S0-AEB-666

“BUT *I* DON’T EAT THAT MUCH”

By the same author

HOW TO GET THINNER ONCE AND FOR ALL

"BUT *I* DON'T EAT THAT MUCH"

A Diet Specialist Answers
His Patients' Questions
on Once-and-for-All Reducing

BY MORTON B. GLENN, M.D.
Past President of the
American College of Nutrition

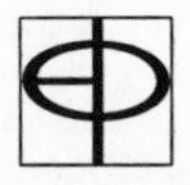

A Sunrise Book
E. P. DUTTON & COMPANY, INC. | NEW YORK | 1974

Library of Congress Cataloging in Publication Data

Glenn, Morton B.
But I don't eat that much

1. Reducing diets. I. Title.
RM222.2.G54 613.2'5 73–79565

First Edition

10 9 8 7 6 5 4 3 2

Published simultaneously in Canada
by Clarke, Irwin & Company Limited, Toronto and Vancouver
ISBN: 0–87690–105–4
Outerbridge & Lazard, a subsidiary of E. P. Dutton & Co., Inc.

To my wife, JUSTINE,
With love and more love.

Contents

Acknowledgments

This book is based primarily on personal experience, and I wish to acknowledge my indebtedness to the many people who have given me this experience: the many physicians who have referred their difficult problems to me, the dieticians and nutritionists who have forced me to find answers to their problems, the many magazine editors who have kept challenging me to find better ways to communicate with the public, and mostly to those thousands of patients who keep saying, "But *I* Don't Eat That Much!"

I also wish to acknowledge the assistance and support of my secretary, Miss Bette Applebaum, and my dietician, Mrs. Suzanne Yachechak, and to my former secretary, Mrs. Francine Paino, for her typing assistance.

And it would not be fair not to acknowledge my wife, who helps in every way.

“But *I* Don’t Eat That Much”

Introduction

Over 20 years ago, I gave my first lecture to the public. The talk was to be 40 minutes in duration, with a 10-minute question-and-answer period, but the question-and-answer period ran considerably beyond the short time allotted for it. During the years that have passed since then, I have consistently spent more of my lecture time in answering questions than in actually lecturing. I have answered the simplest of questions as well as very complex ones; I have also answered outlandish questions and have been amazed at the interest the answers to those questions aroused.

The purpose of this book is twofold: first, to outline my Diet Plan method of weight control. The Diet Plans shown are those used in the treatment of my overweight patients. They are designed to give you a healthy, safe, *proved* method of weight reduction. They are equally designed to give you a style of eating that meets your metabolic and nutritional needs, and one that is appropriate to your cultural (home, occupational, and social) needs, as well as to your psychological requirements. Most of all, they provide for long-term weight control based on sound eating habits. The need to be thinner should not require a change in life style, but rather the creation of an eating style to fit into your life style.

Second, the purpose of this book is to answer your questions—the easy ones, the difficult ones, and possibly some outlandish ones. Both the questions and the answers are based upon my more than 20 years' personal experience in treating problems of weight control. They are the questions and answers that most often have been asked of me.

They span the entire spectrum of my office, clinic, and hospital work, as well as my activities in the fields of public health, community nutrition, clinical research, medical school teaching, and even work in camps for overweight children. In answering the questions I have also drawn upon what is currently being learned in various research laboratories, as well as upon the experiences of colleagues.

Our society has become extremely conscious of weight control. Countless dollars have been spent on it. People have become so concerned with losing weight that it has become a favorite topic of conversation. Some people have become neurotic about it. It has ruined some lives and been the making of others. Diet books fill many shelves in libraries, as do diet foods in supermarkets. Problems of weight control cross every border: national, political, economic, social, racial, and religious. Both sexes and all ages are involved. Concern about weight has become a major problem in the lives of countless people.

It is my theory, proved to the satisfaction of a large number of my patients and readers, that weight control need not be an obsession. I know of no way that one can go to sleep fat and wake up thin. I know of no way to lose weight easily or painlessly. But I do know ways of getting thin and staying thin. If you are like most people, I can tell you how you can do this. What's more, while you're dieting you'll feel at ease, whether you're eating alone, or in a social situation, or in a situation peculiar to your occupation. But it is work—it does require effort and planning. Although it is not easy, at the same time it is not too difficult. It requires some sacrifice, but it is not painful. The method is successful, but *only* if you use it faithfully. If you are serious about your desire to be thinner, if you are mature enough to accept either the full credit for your success or the full blame for your failure, the theories outlined in this book can be a final answer to your weight-control needs. If you want a technique in which the other person does the work, stop now, and give the book to somebody else.

Part One

UNDERSTANDING WEIGHT CONTROL

1

Why People Should Be Thinner

The major reasons for being thinner are of two kinds: medical and emotional. Medically, there is sufficient evidence to show that thinner people tend to have a longer life expectancy and a lower incidence of illness. The evidence for this has been established by the statistics of the insurance companies as well as by the general experience of most physicians. Both diabetes and hypertension (high blood pressure) seem to develop sooner in people who are overweight. Overweight also appears to make these already existing conditions worse.

Surgeons prefer to operate on patients who are leaner, and often tell their overweight patients to lose pounds before an elective operation. Many an individual has had to do this before his surgeon would repair a hernia or remove a gallbladder. Anesthetists feel that thinner people require less anesthesia, and, therefore, that to be overweight means that there is an additional risk when general anesthesia is necessary. Obesity also appears to aggravate disease of the peripheral blood vessels. Most overweight people who suffer from arthritis in their hips, legs, or feet get relief when the weight-bearing joints have less weight to carry. Pregnancy is both safer and easier in the nonoverweight woman. The number of medical conditions aggravated by excessive weight is endless. In addition, there are many conditions where overweight, although not a primary cause of increased death rates, may well be a secondary or tertiary cause. An example of this is the obesity that aggravates, or hastens the development of, high blood pressure or diabetes. These diseases, in turn, are causative or worsening factors in the development of arteriosclerosis (hardening of the arteries), which in its turn causes heart attacks, angina pectoris, and strokes. Thus, overweight must be considered a predisposing factor in the earlier deaths and incapacitation that overtake many people.

A second major reason why people should be thinner is the important emotional role that slimness plays in the lives of so many individuals. Our culture has put a premium on being thin that is out of all proportion to its medical importance. Our society has made a moral issue of thinness, or at least certain classes of it have done so. I personally deplore those elements in our society that are responsible for this value judgment, and feel sorry for the many overweight people who must live under such social standards. Inasmuch as society says it is better to be thinner, however, the overweight individual is usually happier about himself after he has reduced and makes a thin appearance. There is a definite emotional asset to having a good image of oneself.

To continue our discussion of why it is important to control our weight, let us turn now to the questions most often asked on this subject by my patients and others who are interested in reducing their weight.

Is it true that fat people have more trouble getting into college or getting a job?

Yes, it is true. The employer or interviewer often feels some innate prejudice against overweight persons. Our society has always put a premium on appearance and, as mentioned previously, our culture regards the thinner man or woman as better looking than the fatter person. Hence, the thinner individual is often looked upon more favorably by interviewers than is his or her fatter competitor. If an interviewer values self-discipline as an important job requirement, he may feel that the overweight individual is possibly less well disciplined than he should be. There is certainly no difference in the intelligence quotients (I.Q.) of fat people and slim people.

Why are overweight people "so jolly"?

That statement is really incorrect. Overweight people are no more or less jolly than anybody else. Many overweight people, however, are very sensitive and defensive about their appearance, and do their best to direct the conversation so as to draw attention to areas other than their overweight. If they control the conversation, they can divert it away from their appearance. Occasionally, they make humorous references to their looks. It doesn't hurt as much for them to do so as it does when someone else comments on their weight.

Why are fat people the first to arrive at a party? Why are they always so prompt?

Frankly, they do it for safety. Extremely overweight people are worried that if they arrive at a party late they will be trapped into sitting in a chair that is not strong enough for them and then suffer the embarrassing risk of breaking the chair—or standing up when everybody else is sitting.

Whenever I mention breaking chairs, I think of an incident that happened in my office. Though some of my patients may be only a few pounds overweight, some are considerably more than that. The office chairs I use are standard chairs, but are picked for nonobtrusive sturdiness, and a few have some extra, hidden supports. So the only chair that ever broke in my office was mine! And I am of normal weight! It was an embarrassing moment!

2

Why People Are Overweight

My experience with many thousands of patients has taught me that overweight people want to know more about their problem. They want to know the whys and wherefores of weight control. They want to know why what is being done for them in a weight-reduction program will work successfully. There is no need for blind compliance with the old-fashioned attitude, "Do what I tell you, and don't ask questions." In this chapter I shall answer a series of questions that should give the reducer the knowledge and insight necessary for his understanding of overweight and its causes. Unless the dieter understands these things, unless he has an intelligent approach to weight reduction, long-term success cannot be expected.

METABOLISM AND CALORIES

What is the difference between obesity and overweight?

There is much confusion and misunderstanding over the meaning of the terms *obesity* and *overweight*. Obesity is defined as that state in which one is at least 15 to 20 percent over one's desirable weight as a result of fat accumulation. This means that a girl who should weigh 110 pounds, but weighs 135 pounds, is obese! If this is insulting to some readers, I am sorry, but obesity is not a moral judgment, rather it's an anatomical and pathological physical description. Obesity results from an excessive accumulation of fat. *All* obese people are overweight, but not all overweight persons are obese. If one is less than 15 to 20 percent overweight, he is not considered obese.

If you have unusual muscle development (as does the professional weight lifter) you may be overweight, but not obese. If you have a serious water-retention problem (as with severe kidney or heart disease) you may also be overweight without being obese. The countless women who talk about having a water-retention problem, particularly premenstrually or when they are taking birth control pills, or those women going through menopause, are not truly overweight because of the water retention. They may be uncomfortable because of it, and I have known women's weight to go up as much as 10 pounds in these circumstances, but in the absence of severe illness (of the heart, kidneys, or liver, or from protein deficiency, etc.) I have never seen a woman who was significantly overweight *because of* water retention. Most overweight is a consequence of excessive fat deposition, and, therefore, throughout this book I often use the term *overweight* instead of *obesity*. In the vast majority of circumstances, the difference between overweight and obesity is merely one of degree.

What is metabolism, and what does it have to do with weight control and calories?

Metabolism is the sum of all of the body's activities that go into both the building of and the breaking down and destruction of tissue. It is the process by which energy is made available for all of life's needs, from the ingestion of food to the maintenance of essential chemical processes, the performance of muscular activity, and the final elimination of wastes. The amount of energy used in these processes is measured in calories. The term *calorie* is simply a measure of heat expenditure, which in terms of the body is roughly a measure of *work*.*

All the work that the human body does in its living can be measured by the calorie (or the joule). All the work expended in internal activities (the heart pumping, the digestive processes, growing, the respiratory processes and so on), as well as the external activities (walking, talking, running, working, bending, playing, and the like) can

* There is a movement to replace "calorie" with a more precise term, "the *joule*," but I believe this substitution of terms is a long time off. I shall not be surprised, however, if in the constant quest for innovative diets, someone comes up with a new "joule diet." This will, of course, be built around the same calorie concepts, but under a new title.

be measured in calories. All this work requires fuel, which is the food we consume. Food can also be measured by the energy it supplies in terms of calories. When the amount of fuel we consume contains the same number of calories we expend for our internal and external activities, we are said to be in *caloric balance* and our weight remains the same. If we expend more calories than we consume, as in extra physical effort or by taking in less food as in dieting, we are in *negative caloric balance* and must lose weight. Conversely, if we consume more calories than we expend, by either eating more or performing less activity, we go into a *positive caloric balance* and gain weight.

This concept was first recognized by the French chemist Lavoisier in the late eighteenth century. No refutation of this principle has yet stood the test of time. Long-term weight control is totally dependent upon this equation.

What controls metabolism?

As already explained, we may think of metabolism as the sum of the body's activities related to the intake and expenditure of energy. The rate of this activity is determined by need; thus, the body uses more energy when it is running than when sitting, and more energy when it has a fever than when at normal temperature.

The basic rate of energy exchange, *metabolism,* in the body is controlled by the thyroid gland. Individuals with underactive thyroids use up fewer calories than normal. This condition is called *hypothyroidism.* The internal and external activities of such individuals are somewhat slowed and they are usually overweight. People with overactive thyroids (*hyperthyroidism*) are in the reverse condition. Their activities are all quickened and they tend to be thin. When anyone develops hyperthyroidism, he usually loses weight.

Does being overweight mean one has a metabolic problem? What is the relationship of overweight to metabolism?

No, being overweight does not indicate that there is a metabolic problem. The experience of innumerable medical researchers, countless specialists in nutrition, and hosts of experts in metabolic diseases indicates that overweight is nearly always the result of a positive caloric balance (the intake of more calories than are expended) and not of a metabolic imbalance. In my office practice and in my clinics, I have always used the most modern laboratory techniques available to test for metabolic imbalances, and it is truly most uncommon to find one. Occasionally, I even find an overactive thyroid in a patient who is overweight. Overweight is seldom the result of a metabolic defect. The starvation in many parts of the world, the weight loss suffered by inmates of prison camps or after prolonged food deprivation (as is seen in people lost in the woods, or in shipwreck survivors) is dramatic proof of the primary role of the caloric equation in overweight.

What is a "sluggish thyroid"?

One of the most common diagnoses formerly made in patients who were overweight was that they had a "low normal thyroid." This was quickly interpreted to mean a "sluggish thyroid," and suddenly there seemed to be justification for the use of thyroid medication on the patient. Modern medicine no longer considers sluggish metabolism or sluggish thyroid as a valid diagnosis. If a person truly has an underactive thyroid, his trouble should be diagnosed as hypothyroidism, and treated appropriately. The term *sluggish thyroid* is outdated and passing into disuse.

Today, a variety of tests are available for the diagnosis of thyroid diseases. Most of the newer tests involve radioisotope techniques. Some are quite complicated and can be done accurately only in a few highly specialized medical laboratories, whereas others can be carried out satisfactorily even in smaller laboratories. These tests occasionally give inconsistent results; they are often affected by other factors, including other medications such as birth control preparations and over-the-counter common cold medications. Consequently, these tests have to be interpreted with great care.

Even when these tests indicate that the thyroid is functioning normally, some physicians feel that the overweight individual benefits by the use of one of the new thyroid medications. I am not in agreement, except in the rarest of circumstances, and find reports in the medical literature very unconvincing. In my opinion, unless one has a definitely underactive thyroid gland, there is no need for, or benefit to be derived from, thyroid medication. In fact, it is well known that in people with normal thyroids, medically known as being *euthyroid,* the addition of thyroid medication will result in the body producing less of its own thyroid hormone. An excessive use of thyroid medication can result in severe toxic effects, including abnormal cardiac rhythms that can lead to death.

Dr. Marcus A. Rothschild, who is Chief of the Nuclear Medicine Service of the New York Veterans Administration Hospital and Professor of Medicine at New York University School of Medicine, states emphatically that "there is little basis upon which to blame obesity on altered thyroid function." In his experience, he states, very few patients actually suffering from hypothyroidism (underactive thyroids) have been obese.

Why do some physicians say that obesity is a result of faulty carbohydrate metabolism?

I think this is usually erroneous, and is putting the cart before the horse. When a person becomes obese, there is considerable stress on his carbohydrate metabolism mechanism, and when tested, his glucose tolerance is shown to be abnormal. Almost any effective dieting technique, regardless of the amount of carbohydrate taken in, will improve the results of his glucose tolerance test if there is weight loss. The abnormal glucose tolerance is usually the result of, not the cause of, the abnormal caloric overload in obese individuals. Some of the research work that has been done on markedly obese people (these are the people most likely to be hospitalized in metabolic wards) have shown some abnormal metabolic events, but I do not feel it is meaningful to assume the same mechanism holds good for an individual 20 pounds overweight as for one who is 200 pounds overweight.

Should an overweight person have a metabolic evaluation?

A good diagnostician must be a pessimist. He must suspect everything. And, in all fairness, it would not be good medicine not to do a metabolic evaluation. On the other hand, as previously mentioned, the discovery of metabolic defects as a cause of overweight is truly rare.

Can other glands or metabolic diseases be the cause of obesity?

These are truly rare conditions. The hormones produced by one gland usually affect the performance of other glands. Overweight can be seen in glandular diseases, but obesity is often only a minor symptom of these diseases, and other symptoms will help the physician to make an appropriate diagnosis. Rare diseases of the brain may cause obesity, but in the experience of most physicians these diseases are read about in what are called "unusual case reports," but are never seen.

How do you get to be overweight?

By eating too much, by eating more than your body needs. The trouble may lie in excessive quantity or in the incorrect selection of high-calorie foods. During World War II, no one ever came out of a concentration camp fat unless he had some unusual way of obtaining extra rations.

Why do you get fatter as you get older?

As you get older, the body appears to get somewhat more efficient in its utilization of calories, apparently burning less for a given activity (though some new research is beginning to dispute this). There is less physical exercise usually: fewer sports activities are undertaken, you are more likely to ride than walk, and so on. Thus, you begin to expend fewer calories. At the same time, the older you are, the more set in your ways you become, and the less likelihood there is of your eating less to adjust to the lessened caloric output. Increased affluence also makes you more susceptible to richer food and thus increases the caloric intake even more.

Why can some people eat everything and not gain weight, while others seem to gain weight just by looking at food?

Probably this question has been asked of physicians, nutritionists, and dieticians more than any other. I remember once giving a lecture to a group of psychoanalysts and expecting a whole series of challenges to my psychological theories inasmuch as I am not a psychiatrist. Instead, the first question asked was this one.

In studies done in metabolic wards, when a number of patients were placed on identical diets, it was found that people burn up their calories or rather expend their energy in the same manner as other people of about the same height, weight, and age. Some of the reasons why some people gain or lose weight more quickly than others are that taller people will burn up more calories than shorter folk, younger people more than older ones, fatter people more than thin, and more active people more than the less active. If you look at those around you, it is likely that the people on either side of you are higher in some of these categories and lower in others. Truly, there is no group of people who can eat everything and not gain weight.

What is the survivor syndrome?

The bodies of some individuals who have been long-term dieters have probably adapted to the prolonged caloric deprivation by a lowered, possibly more efficient, caloric expenditure. It is possible that some individuals can carry on certain activities with less expenditure of calories than others. This certainly has been seen in prison camps and in lifeboat survivors adrift at sea. In fact, I call it the *survivor syndrome.* Unfortunately, many people who have developed this lowered caloric expenditure often get tired of their constant caloric deprivation, say "to heck with it," and go on an eating binge. The cycle then starts all over. The fact is that most people who say, as so many overweight people do, "But *I* don't eat that much," *are* eating more than they need.

What is the role of exercise in weight control?

We should consider exercise from two points of view: as it relates to the prevention of obesity and to the treatment of obesity. Exercise is extremely important in our present culture in the *prevention of overweight.* We live today in a society where one of our goals is constantly to engage in less and less physical activity. We have mechanical dishwashers and washing machines and power lawnmowers, and I have even seen electric scissors for a person doing a little home sewing. With every diminution of effort, with every ride instead of a walk, with every instance of "let the machine do it," fewer and fewer calories are used. If the amount of calories we take in is not cut down and kept in line with our lessened caloric need, we then become fatter. To avoid fat deposition there must be an absolute balance between caloric intake and output. Lessened physical activity is therefore one of the major reasons why as a society we are today becoming fatter and fatter.

Treating obesity by exercise is another story. I do not feel that exercise is very important in weight reduction, but questions about this will be discussed in Chapter 25, "Exercise, Massage, and Special Aids."

Why do men get potbellies as they get older?

Apparently there is a combination of factors. As one gets older, there is usually less exercise performed, and, consequently, a laxness of the abdominal muscles occurs. More important, there is probably a physiological aging process that is similar to why people get gray hair as they get older. It is sexually related as it is so much more obviously a masculine trait.

I recall reading about an individual who had plastic surgery on his hand. The tissues for the skin graft were transplanted from his abdomen. As he got older and developed an increased amount of abdominal fat, the fat on the back of the hand that had been transplanted also began to increase.

What is the "fat cell" theory?

Fat does not lie about loosely in the body. It is contained in special cells known as *fat cells*. The special purpose of these cells is to hold fat. The body has many specialized cells such as bone cells, muscle cells, and so on. The fat cells have definite cell walls, nuclei, and the ability to carry out certain chemical reactions.

Dr. Jules Hirsch, a medical researcher at Rockefeller University in New York City, together with his colleagues, has demonstrated that certain laboratory animals will have an increased amount of fat cells if they are overfed before weaning; whereas if these animals are not overfed until after weaning, they will have larger cells containing more fat, but they do not develop *more* cells.

This work was extended to humans by Dr. Hirsch, Dr. J. Knittle at Mt. Sinai Medical School, New York City, and Dr. L. Salans at the Dartmouth Medical School. They demonstrated that some overweight humans show an increase in the number of fat cells, whereas others have an increase in the size of the cells, but not in the number of cells. It also appears that the earlier in life one is overfed, the more likely one is to develop an increased number of fat cells.

Does the fat cell theory mean that anyone who has more fat cells is destined to be overweight forever?

No, I do not think so. One of the things demonstrated by Dr. Hirsch and his co-workers is that when an individual is put on a diet, he will lose fat from his fat cells. Individuals with an increased number of fat cells to start with keep their increased number of cells, but they are now empty of, or have less, fat. I like to visualize fat tissue sometimes as if it were a sponge that may either be empty or full of fat, but with its structure otherwise unchanged. There is no convincing evidence that an individual with more fat cells need have any more body fat than an individual with fewer fat cells.

Individuals who have accumulated markedly excessive amounts of fat tissue must also build up extra connective tissue to support the excessive fat cells. When one loses the excessive fat after dieting, some of the connective tissue apparently remains. Possibly this, as well as the empty fat-cell structures, provide a partial explanation for the large abdominal aprons which remain after large weight losses in the excessively obese.

There is much still to be learned about what I call *the anatomy of fat tissue,* and there is great hope for further discoveries in this area. The study of fat cells has opened up new vistas for research that offer much hope for persons who are obese.

THE ROLE OF HEREDITY

Is overweight hereditary?

I question to what extent overweight is hereditary. There are reports of geographically separated twins who become overweight at the same time. Yet, in my practice I have often treated a person who was overweight whose twin was not.

An individual with two fat parents is more likely to be fat than a person with one one fat parent. A person with one fat parent is more likely to be overweight than a person without any fat parents. Does this mean obesity is hereditary? I think not. The only thing that seems to be inherited is where the fat is deposited. Some families have most of their fat in their thighs, or some may have very large buttocks, but I do not think the *amount* of fat is hereditary. I think families are fat because they eat together in a fat fashion. Parents teach eating habits to their children and if the parents are fat, they are probably teaching, if only by example, fat eating habits.

Dr. Jean Mayer of Harvard University has clearly demonstrated a species of mice who have *hereditary obesity*. By this it is meant that when given free choice of food, they will eat more and get fatter than other mice. They can be made to lose weight when given restricted diets. These mice are also characterized by having a high proportion of sterile individuals. The demonstration that a hereditarily obese strain of mice exists does not mean, however, that the same is true of humans. I believe that obesity is "learned" at the dining table, not inherited.

If obesity involves no metabolic or hereditary defect, is it really a disease in the medical sense?

In the sense that it has medical effects, of course it is. But perhaps a better description of overweight and obesity would be that it is a psychosocial disease. It is a disease, or a condition, brought on by a variety of psychological phenomena, conditions, and responses, and is strongly influenced by the social and environmental factors in one's life.

PSYCHOLOGICAL REASONS FOR BEING OVERWEIGHT

What are the psychological factors in becoming overweight?

One could fill an entire book answering this question. Indeed, many books have been written on the subject, but I will try to answer it simply, as one of the many areas of interest in weight reduction.

One would probably need a calculator to add up all the reasons that have been listed for why people overeat, why they continue to overeat, why a person stays fat, or why another may consistently fail at a diet yet suddenly succeed in an additional attempt. Also, there are different combinations of psychological factors. Furthermore, it is my experience that some people overeat for one reason on one day, and for a totally different reason on another day.

Is it psychological if a woman does the best dieting of her life after she announces her engagement, and manages to get to the best possible weight by her wedding day? Is it psychological if a man loses his job, is thwarted in his attempts to get a new one, and suddenly finds it more and more difficult to stick to his diet? Is it psychological when a young woman says, "When I get thinner I will start auditioning for a job as an actress," and by not getting thinner avoids the challenge of the audition? Is it psychological when an overweight teen-ager, who has a poor relationship with a dominating, thin, attractive mother, does poorly on a diet?

People stay fat to avoid situations that they feel they might fail in. Women stay fat to avoid being attractive to men and so avoid getting into difficult or compromising situations. Children use fat to get even with their parents. I cannot count the number of women who get even with their husbands by staying fat. Fat people sometimes get fatter to punish themselves. How many people eat in spite because someone reminds them at the table that they have had enough cake? How many people are so embarrassed by their overeating that they eat only when nobody is looking?

In my experience, the chief reason for overeating is tension, or in today's parlance, what some people would call being uptight. Early in life, many people have learned there is great relief in putting something into their mouths. The mother quickly discovers that a crying baby is controlled by a nipple, whether it contains food or is just an empty pacifier. As the child grows older he sucks his thumb. Later on we see children bite their nails, or put pencils in their mouths. We see adolescent girls twist and put the ends of their hair into their mouths, and chew endless amounts of gum. To this is added the habit of putting extra food or drink into one's mouth. And, of course, the ubiquitous cigarette provides similar relief.

Some of these oral tranquilizers are given up as one grows older. Some are simply replaced by others. Some create habits so ingrained that we indulge them even though there is no tension present at the moment. Thus, not every cigarette is smoked, or nail bitten, or piece of candy eaten because one is tense. One does this by habit; they are pleasurable experiences. However, when a tense moment occurs there is an immediate reversion to one of the oral habits.

One of the interesting observations I have made in my office when interviewing smokers, particularly on the initial visit, is to carefully note what question I have asked when they decide to light a cigarette. Often this is very revealing as to their areas of tension, or what I call *psychic discomfort*.

I am convinced that *over 90 percent* of the overweight patients whom I have seen eat as a manifestation of anxiety or tension. This tension may be associated with depression or even agitation, but it is the tension that is soothed, or tranquilized, or sedated, or, I can even say, narcotized by eating. For some people, this oral sedation requires a sweet taste (though by experience a sour taste has the same effect); for others, chewing is the main need; and for others, the fact that anything is in the mouth suffices. Those individuals who smoke, bite their nails, put pencil ends in their mouth, chew gum, or imbibe too much, as well as overeat are obviously much more dependent on oral outlets than the overweight individual who does not bite his nails or chew gum. It is these oral drives that make the individual who gives up smoking eat more, or the one who begins to eat less smoke more or chew more gum.

What are some of the psychological reasons for gaining weight or, in other words, overeating?

There are probably over fifty psychological considerations that I could enumerate, and often more than one are operating at the same time. The most common ones that I find influencing my patients are as follows:

Boredom: There is nothing interesting to do.
Loneliness: Your husband or wife is away.
Annoyance: Your boyfriend should be taking you out, but isn't.
Jealousy: Your co-worker got the promotion.
Anger: You found your car windshield broken.
Guilt: You said something to your husband or wife you regret.
Need for reward: It's time the world was nice to you.
Fatigue: For many people, eating gives psychological relief when one is tired.

You may also eat to get even with a spouse or a parent. You may eat when you are sad, but a severely depressed person usually loses his appetite.

Are there any other significant psychological factors in overeating?

As mentioned earlier, many psychological factors may be involved, but they are beyond the scope of this book. Particularly important is overeating as a device to stay sexually unattractive. I have seen many young girls who are exceptionally careful with make-up, hair-dos, manicuring, and the other elements of good grooming, who are really doing this to maintain status with other girls in their peer group, while by being fat they really avoid the ultimate confrontation with boys. Unfortunately for some, this goes well beyond the adolescent years. Fat is a great insulator. It can be used to separate you from those around you very effectively. Very often this fat becomes the only protection a girl has against the prodding of a parent who wants her daughter to be more active socially. On the other hand, some parents—particularly mothers of boys—make a practice of giving lip service to wanting their children slim, but are subconsciously encouraging their fatness. (This is discussed further below.)

Another important psychological factor in overeating is motivating those people who have deep-seated resentments against someone close to them, such as a spouse or a parent, and who use being fat as a weapon against their kinfolk. Thus, the child who is very angry at a parent often demonstrates this anger by doing something his parent would not like. In some families thinness is so important that its avoidance becomes a perfect tool to "get even."

Many people withhold sex on the pretext that they are too tired, too busy, have to get up early the next day, and the like as a method of showing displeasure at the actions of a spouse. In the same manner, when it is very important to a man for his wife to be thin, she may use fatness as a method of showing her anger and annoyance with him.

Obviously using fatness as a weapon is a little like kicking someone hard enough to break your own ankle. No matter how much the other person deserves the kick, it was not worth having your foot in a plaster cast for six weeks!

What is the "fatty game"?

This is one of the psychological games that fat families play. The main players in this game are an overweight mother, a father who may or may not be overweight, and an overweight child. The overweight mother will tell the child, "I wish you would stop eating the way you do. Your weight is much higher than it should be. You'll just have to be more careful about overeating."

Then the father will ask the mother, "Why did you get cake at the market?"

And the mother will answer, "Well, after all, it's his birthday, and I think he is entitled to some cake on his birthday. He can start his diet tomorrow."

Tomorrow there will, of course, be some leftover cake and somebody will say, "Well we shouldn't waste it." Obviously, these diets never start, but everybody is getting angry at everybody else, and blaming each other. Very often the mother who is telling her child to get thinner is really keeping him fat by constantly supplying too much food. She is insuring his dependency on her maternalism.

A few years ago I saw a variation of this in an older individual when a young woman, Joan L., came to me, encouraged by, and with some pressure from, her mother. Joan was about 23 years old, a schoolteacher, and lived alone in an apartment not far from her mother. Joan's mother was very close to her, saw her at least four times a week, and insisted that when her daughter came home from school she should call her to let her "know that she was safe." Joan's mother also would often supply her daughter with food. Since she had a key to Joan's apartment, she would simply buy what she thought was appropriate and leave it there. Joan's mother stocked the larder with a large supply of cookies and candy in case Joan had company.

Joan made slower progress with her dieting than she should have, and with the passage of time it became obvious that she was overly dependent upon her mother. She accepted as a matter of course all the extra little things her mother would do for her, and the older woman felt warmly rewarded by Joan's closeness. I tried to show Joan that though closeness was nice, it would be better for her to become a little more independent. The more I encouraged this independence, the more Joan's mother began to discourage her daughter from seeing me. The older woman recognized me as a threat to her. At this point it was obvious that as much as Joan's mother did for her, and close as the mother and daughter were, it was not a healthy relationship. On Joan's very first visit to my office, when I take the initial hour-long patient history, her mother had felt quite insulted when I insisted on seeing Joan without her in the room. I was reminded of this when one day I saw Joan, quite fat, walking with her mother into a gourmet food shop. Joan would never really work out her weight problem until she developed a healthier, more mature relationship with her mother.

Are overweight people psychologically different from nonoverweight or thin people?

If one looks carefully one can see the very same traits in thin people as in overweight people. The major difference is simply that overweight people may express some of their psychological needs in the form of eating. On the other hand, thin people sometimes do the same thing but, as the mathematicians might say, they do it with a minus sign instead of a plus sign. Thus, extreme nervousness in some persons is handled by an increase in appetite, whereas in others it causes a loss of appetite.

To be fat does not mean that one need be ungraceful, and to be thin need not mean that one is weak. In the same way, there is not necessarily any difference between the overweight and nonoverweight person in intelligence, emotions, or any other psychological traits. Fat people and thin people can be equally sad, happy, funny, lonely, or friendly.

Is it true that overweight people are really hiding from other people by being fat?

Some psychiatrists think so. By being fat such persons have a tendency to avoid going out, using the excuse that they do not look well, so in effect the overweight person uses his weight as an insulator against the world. Of course the paradox of the situation is that the fatter people get the more obvious they are, and they receive that much more attention by the mere state of their appearance.

What is the "raincoat brigade"?

Some time ago a magazine writer was interviewing me for an article about overweight women. I suggested that she use in her story the term, *the raincoat brigade.* I was referring to a whole group of women who are so conscious of their overweight that they try to hide it in any manner possible. Many of these women wear lightweight raincoats in the summer, thinking they are hiding their fatness. It almost goes with out saying that if one sees a woman on a clear, beautiful, hot day wearing a lightweight raincoat, she is trying to hide her excess weight.

Does being fat mean you are neurotic?

I like to think of neurosis as a state in which one's emotional needs and responses reach the point where they interfere with a normal participation in and enjoyment of life. If one feels, for example, that because of being overweight his appearance is such that he refuses to go to a party, that is neurotic. If one feels that he is too fat to accept a date, that is neurotic. If you are fat, ask yourself to what extent you allow it to interfere with your life style. You can then judge to what extent your fatness has involved you in neurosis.

I had one patient who told me that the only trouble with being fat was that "his neurosis was showing." Perhaps in his case it was. Rather than asking whether being fat means one is neurotic, it is probably more pertinent to ask to what extent any excessive eating is psychologically significant.

3

Who Should Diet —and Who Should Not

Anyone who is obese, with the occasional exceptions noted below, would probably benefit medically from weight reduction. For some, the question is not whether they should diet, but when is the best time to diet. The degree of overweight clearly affects the decision also. Slightly overweight people must decide for themselves whether they would rather put up with a larger dress or suit size, or the discipline of a good diet.

The following questions are the one I am most often asked in terms of who should and who should not diet.

Does everybody want to be thin? Does everybody who is overweight want to lose weight?

In our society, most overweight people say they wish they were not overweight. A few say that they are perfectly happy to be the way they are. Some of them may be, but some may not be, regardless of what they say. Few people like to admit that they are unhappy, particularly if they have control over this unhappiness. For some overweight people, to be overweight serves a psychological need. Often they are only deluding themselves into believing that they would like to be thinner, not realizing that unconsciously they are choosing to be fatter rather than thinner. In the long run, most people who say they wish to be thinner and do not get thinner are unconsciously indicating that they do not want to get thinner. *Getting thin is a matter of choice—the individual's own choice.* The physician's role can only be one of helping the individual to achieve his true goal. If the goal, no matter how unconscious, is not to get thinner, there is little likelihood that any weight-control program, regardless of method, will be successful. If one does get thin under these circumstances, it is most likely that he will regain the weight.

Should everybody be thin?

No, not everybody is better off being thin. Certainly, there is sufficient medical evidence to indicate that people in general are healthier when they are thinner. I use the words *in general* because there are special circumstances in which people have other medical conditions that may make it more advisable to have some extra weight. If you are not certain whether it is medically advisable for you to lose weight, consult your physician and allow him to advise you.

Is there anyone who should not diet?

Yes. Such individuals include the following:

1. People who are too thin
2. People who have recently stopped smoking
3. People who have other medical problems
4. People who have emotional problems

It always comes as a surprise to overweight people that persons who are very thin often want to become thinner. This is a result of the thinness obsession of so many people. I see it mostly in ballet dancers and in some of the fashion models. I do not think that any ballet master ever thinks that his dancers are thin enough, but in reality—except for a few dancers who have become careless about their eating habits, or who have been incapacitated by an injury—it is unusual to encounter an overweight ballet dancer.

In another situation, I have a patient who is doing very well on her diet. Her very thin boyfriend, who lives with her, feels that it is important for them to share equally in all things. Accordingly, he is following her diet and becoming too thin. My patient is becoming healthier and more attractive, her boyfriend the reverse!

Another group of people who should not diet are those who have given up smoking very recently. In my experience, the vast majority of persons who go on a stringent weight-reduction program simultaneously with giving up smoking usually fail at both. If you were a heavy smoker, *wait until you are reasonably certain you will not go back to smoking* before starting to diet. Be careful in your eating, but do not start an intensive diet program too early. If you smoked one pack a day, wait at least one month before starting an intensive diet program, and if you smoked two or more packs wait at least three months.

Any individual with a specific medical disease, or who is on special medication, should not diet without the approval of his physician. Individuals with ulcers, food allergies, or colitis, or diabetics on insulin should not start any weight-reduction diet without first consulting their doctor. In general, if you are not 100 percent healthy, do not diet—do not use any diet—without your physician's permission. Show your doctor the diet you intend to follow, and get his specific approval of it before starting.

For persons with certain types of emotional problems and under heavy stress, eating may be the only tranquilizer that allows them to function without having a serious breakdown. I recently had a patient whose son was dying from a brain tumor. The son's wife was working to support the family and my patient was trying to keep the home together, but the deterioration of her world was getting her down. This was not the time for her to diet.

For some people, the trials and tribulations of dieting and the concept of self-denial in the area of food may be so difficult, so trying, so impossible to cope with psychologically that they may truly be better off not dieting. The medical advantages simply may not compensate for the psychological problems endured by some dieters. This is particularly true in periods of anxiety. There is no question that these periods of anxiety can occur to the extent where they become overwhelming, and take precedence over other aspects of one's life. I recall one patient whose husband had just asked her for a divorce a week after she had started her diet. Her weight did not appear to be in any way related to her husband's attitude toward her, but her anxieties were so great that I felt that this was not the time for her to diet. On the other hand, not long ago a young woman patient who was recently separated from her husband told me in a most determined manner that if she had to reenter the "singles" world, she had better look her very best.

I strongly believe, however, that the majority of overweight people do better both physically and emotionally when they are no longer overweight, and that more often than not they are able to cope with the psychological problems that may be caused by dieting.

Should people be forced into dieting?

I do not think anyone *can* be forced into dieting. One can be encouraged, cajoled, even tricked, but never forced. One can reason with a person who should lose weight, and hope to convince him or her to make the decision to start a weight-control program, but they cannot be forced. I have been told many stories about parents who claim to have forced children to lose weight, but I have never seen any statistics on how long the weight loss has persisted.

Sometimes I have seen patients create a whole set of excuses in order to avoid dieting, and then feel their consciences were free if they could convince their physician to tell them not to diet. Some years ago, a rather well-known Hollywood actor was referred to me by his doctor. The man said he was desperate to lose weight because unless he did he would lose a major part in a forthcoming picture. After telling me his plight, he then began to recite a dozen reasons, none of them very good, why he would probably fail at dieting and why I should refuse to accept him as a patient. After hearing his long and somewhat dramatically told story, I told him that I thought he was right, that he would probably fail at dieting, and it was pointless for him to start. But I also said that the real reason he should not begin to diet was that he did not want to diet, and the whole effort would be a waste of time. He became so upset that he did a complete about-face, deciding he did want to diet, and I started him on a program on which he lost a very large amount of weight. Unfortunately, the passage of time showed that he had a major problem with alcohol, and this was making his eating needs secondary to his drinking needs. I no longer see mention of him in the newspapers, so I do not know the final outcome.

How do you get a child to want to lose weight?

This is often a difficult task, primarily for the reason that most children do not see any really good reason to lose weight. Life treats them well whether they are thin or fat. Usually their biggest reason for reducing is simply that they are being pressured by their parents. Occasionally, children are called names by their friends, such as "Fatty," "Tubby," and others even less kind. Children can, of course, be rather cruel to one another. Besides this name-calling, the overweight child's mother often complains about the difficulty of getting clothes to fit him.

In trying to motivate a child to lose weight, one should stress the fact that if he does, the name-calling will stop. Second, we point out to little girls the importance of looking well, and remind them that anyone who is thinner can expect to look better. Boys are often quite responsive to the argument that if they weighed less they would have less fat and more muscle and would therefore be stronger, as well as quicker, in sports.

Both boys and girls also respond when I tell them that they might do better in school if they were less fat. They would concentrate more on their work than on eating. A wonderful device for influencing a little girl to reduce is to give her a full-length mirror for her own room. Girls learn very early to look at themselves in the mirror and to groom themselves. So get your child a full-length mirror; it may be very helpful to her.

From the point of view of life expectancy, is it worse to be a smoker or to be overweight?

The statistics seem to indicate that smoking is worse than being overweight. I suggested above that people who wish to give up smoking should do so first, and postpone starting a diet program until they are confident they will not go back to smoking. In the long run it is easier to control smoking than eating, primarily because smoking is an all-or-nothing situation; that is, you can exist without ever smoking again. Eating, on the other hand, is something that you must do in moderation for the rest of your life. Dealing with things in moderation is always considerably more difficult than dealing with an all-or-nothing situation.

If one is overweight, there is a strong probability that it would be advantageous to lose weight. There may be extenuating physical or emotional circumstances that do mitigate against dieting for some people at certain times and in certain circumstances. The degree of overweight should play the largest role in determining whether you should diet, together with the degree of discomfort resulting from being overweight. Incidentally, it is very common for an overweight person at the beginning of a diet to say he feels absolutely perfect, but it is equally common for this same person to forget that he said this and after a period of time on a good diet to say, "You can't imagine how much better I feel since I've lost weight."

4

How Much Should You Weigh?

There is no simple answer to this question. Many factors must be taken into consideration. The most important question is what weight would provide optimal health. All the weight goals given in this book are those that are considered to be medically desirable. For convenience I have included on pages 31–32 a weight chart that gives what I consider to be maximum weights, or, in other words, the highest weights for optimal health. These weights are based on heights without shoes and on frame sizes (see pages 33–34 on determining one's frame size).

A second consideration is what weight is culturally acceptable. In other words, within your world—within the group of people you associate with—what weight is considered to be appropriate? Some people live in a milieu where weight is commonly close to the upper limits of the medically correct level, and others in circles where weights are much nearer to the lower level. As an example, for the high-fashion world the weights given in these charts are considerably higher than what is considered "normal" weight.

A third determinant is what I call the body-image concept. Most of us have an image of how we would like to look—very slim or very curvaceous, and so forth. Obviously our bone structure and our general build may prevent us from looking the way we would like to look. Very large-boned persons may look thin but they could never look petite, any more than a person with an extremely small-boned structure could look robust.

Still another factor in determining correct weight is fat distribution as it relates to body proportions. Some people appear to have more fat on the upper half of their body, while in others it appears on the lower half. If losing weight aggravates an unwanted fat distribution, one often must make some compromise in one's weight goal. Many women complain that in order to lose more weight in their hips and thighs, they would lose too much in the face and bust. This is a decision each woman must make for herself.

Probably the best single method of determining one's best weight,* and this is one that I use with my patients, is measuring by means of skin calipers. These are measurements of subcutaneous fat (fat under the skin) in various parts of the body, made with a special instrument called a skin-thickness caliper. Actually, this instrument measures the thickness of skin and fat. Skin-thickness calipers are not used often today, except in research institutions. They have certainly been used extensively in nutritional surveys throughout the world, but for some reason are neglected by many physicians. I find them indispensable and the best single determinant of what an individual's optimal weight is.

To sum up, you must put together all the factors to establish your "correct weight." You are much better off not concerning yourself with what you should weigh at the beginning of your diet, but rather saving that decision for when you are nearer to a probable goal. If you are tired of dieting, or are suddenly reaching a plateau on your diet, and therefore rationalize that you have achieved a satisfactory goal, stop and look in a mirror! Decide on your goal honestly and realistically. Too many stop their dieting prematurely. Do not be lazy with just a few pounds to go.

Are there different kinds of height-weight charts?

There are two basic kinds of height-weight charts. One type is called the *average weight chart*. It simply gives the average weights of a large group of people of different heights. All that these charts really show you is how you compare with the rest of the group. The groups whose heights and weights are charted are usually a countrywide sampling. Standards do vary from country to country.

A more commonly used type of chart is the *desirable weight chart*

---

* In medical research laboratories, obesity measurements are often taken in terms of lean body mass determinations. This is a determination that basically measures all nonfatty tissue. These determinations are made by underwater weighing, and by isotope-dilution studies. They are too complicated and too expensive for general clinical use.

or *ideal weight chart,* as it is sometimes less accurately labeled. These charts have been constructed by insurance companies, based on weights and longevity, and the word *desirable* refers to life expectancy. These charts show the weights at which, statistically, an individual is most likely to live the longest, all other things being equal. Desirable weight charts are based on height, sex, and body frame, but not on age: All people 25 years of age or older are grouped together. Those younger than 25 simply subtract a pound for each year under 25.

In reading a chart, be careful to note whether it gives weight with or without clothing, or weight with or without shoes. Most of the standard charts today are based on weights with shoes and with clothing (but without jackets). Though desirable weights are given in the form of a range from high to low, I have found it easier to use an average from these ranges. The charts which follow show what I consider to be the maximum desirable weights—the weights below which people are most likely to have the longest life expectancy.

MAXIMUM WEIGHT FOR WOMEN*

Weight Is Without Clothes†
Height Is Without Shoes

HEIGHT	SMALL FRAME‡	AVERAGE FRAME	LARGE FRAME
4′8″	95	104	116
4′9″	98	107	119
4′10″	101	110	122
4′11″	104	113	125
5′0″	107	116	128
5′1″	110	119	131
5′2″	113	123	135
5′3″	116	127	139
5′4″	120	132	143
5′5″	124	136	147
5′6″	128	140	151
5′7″	132	144	155
5′8″	137	148	160
5′9″	141	152	165
5′10″	145	156	170
5′11″	149	160	175
6′0″	153	165	181

* Adapted from Metropolitan Life Insurance Co. For women between 18 and 25, subtract 1 pound for each year under 25.

† To determine weight with shoes and clothes, add 2 to 5 pounds.

‡ For determining your frame, see pages 33–34.

MAXIMUM WEIGHT FOR MEN*

Weight Is Without Clothes†
Height Is Without Shoes

HEIGHT	SMALL FRAME‡	AVERAGE FRAME	LARGE FRAME
5′1″	116	125	137
5′2″	119	129	140
5′3″	122	132	144
5′4″	125	135	148
5′5″	129	139	152
5′6″	133	143	157
5′7″	137	148	162
5′8″	141	152	166
5′9″	146	156	170
5′10″	150	161	175
5′11″	154	166	180
6′0″	158	171	185
6′1″	163	176	190
6′2″	167	181	195
6′3″	171	186	200
6′4″	175	191	205

* Adapted from Metropolitan Life Insurance Co.
† To determine weight with shoes and clothes, add 3 to 6 pounds.
‡ For determining your frame, see pages 33–34.

Are there exceptions to these charts?

In general, when you make an exception, this exception should be by choosing a lower weight rather than a higher weight. But this may be a decision to consult your physician about, and it is hoped he is not a fat physician.

What if some of the weights on the charts seem ridiculously low?

If they seem ridiculously low, do not get that thin. When I discuss a final weight with a patient, occasionally one will make the statement, "I haven't weighed that little since I was growing." I must admit that I have a fairly stock answer to this. I always compare it to a situation in which I ask my patient, if you have never had money before, does that mean that you would refuse to get rich now? A chart weight is usually valid. If it is too low for you, you have one perfect recourse: You can always regain the weight. Once you have lost a large amount of weight, you should reassess your frame. This, in turn, may suggest a reevaluation of what your weight should be.

A good standard for most married women is the weight at which they got married. And for many men, a good standard is their weight when they were in the armed forces, that usually being associated with a period of top physical condition.

How do I tell my correct frame?

This is not always easy, primarily because there have never been any absolute standards to determine precisely what a large, medium, or small frame is, or how to measure it. The term *frame* refers basically to bone size and muscle development. "Wide hips" denotes a "female" type of pelvis, not a wide frame. When we say someone has "broad shoulders," we occasionally mean that his shoulders are fat rather than well muscled. So far as the charts are concerned, however, being fat does not mean that one has a large frame any more than being skinny means that one has a small frame.

In my experience, the best determinant of body frame is wrist size. Are the wrists very large, medium, or really very small? There are no specific measurements for these sizes; it is a matter of interpretive judgment. The next best measurement is the width of one's foot. This is best told by one's shoe width and is probably a better determinant than shoe length, which usually is more consistent with body height than with frame. Most people with wide feet have large frames, whereas those with narrow feet have small frames, and, of course, the middle sizes lie in between. Another way to determine frame is one's hand size. (Most women know their glove sizes, though very few men do.) The same rules would hold here as for wrist size: A very large hand tends to go with a large frame and a small hand with a small frame. In men, a very good indication of frame is the size of the head. Today few men know their hat size. In general, a hat size of about 7½ would be consistent with a large frame, and a hat size of 7 or less tends to go with a small frame. Those in between go with a middle-sized frame. Sometimes one will arrive at the answer that one's frame is somewhere between a small and medium, or between medium and large. There may not be a precise answer regarding your frame size. Obviously, however, most people fall into the category of having medium-sized frames.

The truest evaluation of frame size is obtained if one can use a combination of all these determinants. The best time to determine one's frame size is when most of the excess fat has been lost! A much better judgment can then be made. Hold off making this determination *until* you are close to a good weight.

Part Two

THE TECHNIQUES OF WEIGHT CONTROL

5

The Diet Plans

We are now almost at the point where we can turn from the goals of weight control to the techniques of achieving these goals. First, however, we must really ask ourselves the basic question: If overweight is primarily a psychosocial disease, is diet the answer to weight control?

If we take this question in its most literal sense, the answer is no! But diet is the *means of control.* . . . In order to be successful, both the Diet Plan and the dieter must provide certain resources. The dieter must bring to the job two major requisites:

Motivation. Motivation does not mean merely desire, but rather the willingness to do whatever is necessary to accomplish the desire.

Self-discipline. This is out-and-out stick-to-itiveness. Twenty years ago, when we used moral judgments rather than the vocabulary of psychology, self-discipline was called *character.* Whatever one calls it, it is an absolute requirement for success.

On the other hand, the Diet Plan must provide:

1. The proper food education
2. The proper nutrients for good health, and an absence of ill effects
3. The proper caloric deficit to provide an appropriate weight loss without unnecessary and unrealistic deprivation
4. An eating style appropriate to your living style
5. A basis for the development of long-term, good eating patterns

This combination of what you bring to a weight-control program and what the Diet Plan supplies to you will provide successful weight loss without changing your life style. In order to insure the permanence of this weight loss, two additional factors are required:

Insight. Every time you make a purposeful error in dieting—and most errors are really purposeful—you are deliberately choosing not to get thinner. You must ask yourself why. The more closely you examine your attitude, the sooner you will understand the *why* of what you are doing. Obviously, physicians, dieticians, teachers, and many others can assist you in the insight-gaining process, but you will be able to develop much of it yourself if you are willing to do so. Being aware of why you are *miseating* is a requirement in controlling this miseating.

The recognition that you will never be able to go back to your old eating habits. One learns new eating techniques during the diet by the process of dieting. A good diet is basically a restrictive exaggeration of a good eating habit. On achieving the correct weight, one drops the restrictive exaggeration but maintains the eating pattern. This is what becomes the permanent eating habit. Maintaining this eating habit is what keeps the weight off forever. *If you go back to your old eating patterns, you will go back to your old weight.* That is what got you to that weight in the first place. It can get you there again!

One of the most important considerations is the fact that there is no one method, no one diet, no one philosophy of weight reduction that meets all people's needs. The techniques suggested in this book are the methods that have given more *long-term* success than any others used today. Almost any method can be successful briefly, but few have stood the test of time. Those presented here have stood that test longer than any other methods I know.

The Diet Plans which follow also have these advantages: They are healthful methods of weight reduction and will not cause any nutritional deficit. They contain the proper amounts of vitamins and minerals for good health, and are low in saturated fats and cholesterol. They are high in protein so as to provide the best source of body-building substances and to meet the requirements of daily wear and tear on the system. Though moderate in carbohydrates, they supply enough to provide sufficient energy for one's daily activities, and enough fuel sources so that the body will not burn its protein resources unnecessarily. (This is what may happen on a low-carbohydrate diet.) Finally, they are designed to fit into one's usual life style: There is no need to change one's style of life simply because an eating habit is changed.

These diets may not be for you; but then they may be. Show them to your physician if you have any doubts. The biggest complaint from my patients about these diets is that there is too much to eat. Not a bad complaint for a diet! Follow them if you are overweight. You stand a very good chance of being helped. But above all, do not modify them or eat less than the diet calls for.

I am reminded of a patient of mine, Mrs. J. L., a 38-year-old, highly successful department store executive. It was easy to see why she was successful. She was efficient in her manner, very punctual, never afraid to say what she meant, and most precise in her choice of words. After I'd taken her history, she proceeded to tell me all the things "that work and do not work" for her in dieting, and requested that I please adjust her diet to these requirements. I told her quite bluntly that I would not accept her rules. I would concede to any religious food restrictions, any food allergies, or any violent food dislikes but the rules had to be mine. After all, I explained, her rules had obviously kept her fat, or she would not have come in to see me in the first place. Therefore, I would require that she follow my rules. She resented my arguments, but logically found it difficult to disagree with them. If you wish to follow the dietary programs in this book, *do not change them—do not modify them!* Forget that you know what works best for you and follow what *has* worked for so many others.

Before choosing your particular Diet Plan from among those given below, the following general instructions are important, not only for the diet itself, but also for developing those habits that will allow you to keep your weight under permanent control.

Never eat unless you are seated. Yes, actually sitting down, and preferably using a plate, knife, and fork, even if it is only a fruit snack. You will do less nibbling, less tasting, if you follow this rule. How many times have you stood in front of the refrigerator, or with a cookie jar in hand, tasting what you were going to eat, and never remembering that the food you were tasting was also loaded with calories. If you went to the trouble of putting the food on a plate and sat down with knife, fork, and napkin, the probability is you just would not bother.

Eat more slowly. Eat slower than yesterday, and slower than anyone else you are eating with. Chew longer and more slowly. Actually dawdle, if possible. A physician-patient of mine once told me that he was out on a date with a woman whom he described was "a tiny little thing." He had just begun his diet and was very conscious of everything, and could not help but notice that his date dawdled, drank sips of water, frequently put down her fork while she spoke to him. As he put it, she "took forever." When he tried to use my trick and eat more slowly than she was doing, he found it agonizing at first. Gradually, however, he became accustomed to eating more slowly, recognizing that he would eat less that way, yet feel more satisfied. Incidentally, this doctor-patient lost about 60 pounds, and although it is now 10 years since his diet, he has maintained his weight loss. He gives major credit for his success to the fact that he learned to eat more slowly. *No fast eater can necessarily become a slow eater, but any fast eater can become a slower one!*

Leave something over on your plate. Leave a small amount of every separate food item. Leave over one string bean, a slice of carrot, a wedge of the half grapefruit. The reason for this is to teach yourself better control. *Control* is the key word, not only in dieting, but also in weight maintenance. If you are overweight or trying to avoid becoming overweight, it is not wasteful to leave something over. It is biologically and economically more wasteful to be fat. And the starving children in Asia are not benefited by the fact that you are a member of the Clean Plate Club. Incidentally, leaving something over on your plate is the most difficult thing for dieters to do, in my experience. You will forget this rule. Remind yourself and reremind yourself. It is important.

Do not take tastes while you are cooking or from other's plates. In a restaurant, eat your own food, not your spouse's! That tiny taste will continuously put tiny amounts of extra fat on you. And if you cannot carry your baby's plate from the table to the sink without eating his leftovers, remember that if you act like a garbage can, you will look like one.

Learn to measure food portions correctly. Use a small postage scale at home. A little practice with the scale will make you a very good estimator when you are away from home. For liquid measurements, use a measuring cup.

If you are in doubt about a particular food item, look it up in this book before you eat it. If you are still not sure, do not eat it.

Do not eat in the bedroom. Eating should be restricted to the eating rooms only. This will control careless eating. This should be particularly emphasized with teen-agers.

The Diet Plans that follow are designed specifically for weight control: achieving a desired weight and staying there. Most people should be able to follow them. In my experience, there are few who cannot do so if they are properly motivated. If you are excessively overweight or have any special medical problems, consult with your physician before starting the diet. Let him supervise you.

If you are a vegetarian, or have special religious restrictions, or eat only organic foods the Diet Plans should present no problem.

Before starting your Diet Plan, get yourself a notebook and begin two sets of records. The first will be a weight record. Write down your starting weight. Weigh yourself weekly, not daily. It is too frustrating to see the large variations in daily weights while on a diet, simply as a result of changes in the body's water balance. Keep a record of your weekly weights, your weekly losses, your total loss. Women should also keep a record of the onset of their menstruation, and note whether there is any water-retention pattern.

Women can tell whether there is a water retention pattern by noting whether or not there is a weight increase at the same time each month in relation to their periods. At the time of such gain, there will often be a feeling of bloating, and finger rings may feel quite tight.

The second record that one should keep is a constant record of everything you eat. If you go over it and circle any incorrect items with a colored pencil, it will increase your awareness of dieting mistakes. Also, if you have a record and run into a prolonged plateau problem, you can show it to a physician (or he can refer you to his hospital's dietician) to look for errors that you may not be aware of to account for the plateau.

By following one of the Diet Plans given in this book, you can expect to lose weight at the rate of 100 pounds per year, though actually, of course, few people need to lose that much. Still, these diets are designed for you to lose about 2 pounds per week. Two pounds per week is 100 pounds per year.

Here are some general rules about rate of weight loss:

The fatter you are, the quicker you lose.
The taller you are, the quicker you lose.
The younger you are, the quicker you lose.
The more active you are, the quicker you lose.
The *better* you diet, the quicker you lose.

These Diet Plans have all been tested. All have proved feasible, appropriate, and successful with many patients. Now let us note the rules for diet selection.

HOW TO SELECT THE CORRECT DIET PLAN

In the following pages (44–82) you will find fourteen different diet plans. These have been designed to fit individual requirements according to sex, age, and the number of pounds one needs to lose. The first step, therefore, is to select the particular Diet Plan that fits your individual case. The following directions are for determining which Diet Plan is the right one for you (or for your child if you are selecting a Diet Plan for a young person).

Women (18 years of age and older)

With less than 10 pounds to lose, follow Diet Plan 2.

With 10 to 49 pounds to lose, follow Diet Plan 3.

With 50 to 99 pounds to lose, follow Diet Plan 3A.

With 100 or more pounds to lose, follow Diet Plan 4.

If you are in doubt as to how much you should lose, choose the Diet Plan with the higher number, *not* the lower number.

Teen-aged Girls

With less than 10 pounds to lose, follow Diet Plan 3C.

With 10 to 49 pounds to lose, follow Diet Plan 3D.

With 50 or more pounds to lose, follow Diet Plan 4B.

Preteen Girls

Follow Diet Plan 3E.

Men (20 years of age and older)

With less than 10 pounds to lose, follow Diet Plan 3B.

With 10 to 49 pounds to lose, follow Diet Plan 4.

With 50 to 99 pounds to lose, follow Diet Plan 4A.

With 100 or more pounds to lose, follow Diet Plan 5.

Teen-aged Boys

With less than 50 pounds to lose, and minimal athletic activity, follow Diet Plan 4B.

With less than 50 pounds to lose, and maximum athletic activity, follow Diet Plan 4C.

With 50 or more pounds to lose, follow Diet Plan 5A.

Preteen Boys

Follow Diet Plan 3E.

Modifications for diet selection in special circumstances

If living in college dormitory away from home add a second fruit in the evening.

If you are pregnant and overweight at the start of your diet, or are gaining more than 2½ pounds per month, *and with your doctor's permission:*

1. Do not use Diet 2 (use 3, 3A, or 4)
2. You *must* have the two glasses of milk throughout the pregnancy
3. When you reach the seventh month, if you are on Diet Plan 3 or 3B, change to Diet Plan 4.

If you are involved in excessive physical labor, increase your diet by one number (if you are on Diet Plan 3, go on to Diet Plan 4, etc.).

If you are over 60 years old, or unusually inactive (in a wheelchair, etc.) decrease your diet by one number, for example, if on Diet Plan 3, go to Diet Plan 2; if Diet Plan 2, go to Diet Plan 1, and so forth.

Now that you understand how to select the proper diet for you, here are the Diet Plans themselves.

DIET PLAN 1

BREAKFAST (must be eaten)	NOTES
4 oz. orange, grapefruit, *or* tomato juice, OR 1 orange, OR ½ grapefruit	May use another fruit, but then one fruit during day must be citrus. Juices must be unsweetened.
AND	
1 egg (made without fat)	
OR	
2 oz. cottage cheese *or* 1 oz. farmer cheese	Use diet cottage cheese if available.
OR	
¾ oz. hard cheese	
OR	
2 oz. fish (1 oz. if smoked)	
AND	
1 slice of *thinly* sliced bread	*No* butter or margarine!
OR	
½ cup of cooked cereal OR ½ oz. of dry cereal } with milk from allowance	Dry cereals must be unsugared. If desired, may have 1 oz. of dry cereal, but give up egg or cheese.
AND	
Beverage: tea *or* coffee *or* milk from allowance if desired	Never use milk, cream, or sugar; lemon may be used.
MID-MORNING (if desired—not required)	
Tea, coffee, *or* bouillon	In any amount.
LUNCH (do not skip lunch)	
Clear soup (any amount) *or* 4 oz. tomato juice if desired (these are optional items)	Soup may be hot or cold, but clear enough to see through.
AND	
4 oz. cottage cheese	Preferably diet cottage cheese, but do not worry if it is not.
OR	
1 oz. hard cheese	
OR	
2 eggs	Avoid eating more than four eggs per week.
OR	

DIET PLAN 1 (cont.)

2 oz. meat, fish, shellfish, *or* poultry	Avoid any fish canned in oil.
AND	
All the raw vegetable salad you wish— NO LIMIT!	But avoid raw peas.
AND	
1 slice of bread OR ½ cup cooked vegetable	If available, use thinly sliced bread.
AND	
Beverage	
MID-AFTERNOON (optional)	
Tea, coffee, bouillon, *or* milk from allowance	If still hungry, you may eat raw vegetables freely, and drink a diet soda, *and, if you wish,* eat your evening snack at this time instead of later.
DINNER	
Clear soup *or* 4 oz. tomato juice	
AND	
3 to 4 oz. meat, fish, *or* poultry	Use fish and poultry mostly.
AND	
1 or 2 portions of cooked vegetables, each a ½-cup serving	Never exceed ½ cup per portion; never have a full cup of one vegetable.
AND	
All the raw vegetable salad you desire	Use lemon, vinegar or some dietetic dressings; never use oil.
AND	
Beverage	
Dessert	None, unless you would prefer your evening snack at this time rather than later.

DIET PLAN 1 (cont.)

EVENING (if desired)	
Tea, coffee, *or* milk from allowance	
AND	
1 fruit *or* ¾ oz. hard cheese *or* ¾ oz. of dry cereal with milk from allowance	Measure cereal carefully.

No butter, margarine, oil, mayonnaise, sour or sweet cream, or regular salad dressings

No sugar, honey, jelly, jam, or diet jelly

MILK:

You should have at least one 8-oz. glass of skimmed milk daily. You may have up to two glasses daily.

ICE CREAM:

You may have 4 oz. (liquid-volume measurement, not weight!) of ice cream or ice milk, three or four times a week in place of a dessert or between-meal snack eaten at the time you are giving up the fruit or cheese. In addition, you must give up a glass of milk for the day. Ice milk is not required, but is preferable to ice cream.

MEAT:

Beef, lamb, and pork (very lean cuts only) are restricted to a maximum of three lunches *and* three dinners per week.

If you miss a food item, you may not make up for it by having it later in the day or at another meal. If you have any doubts, *do not eat it!*

DIET PLAN 2

BREAKFAST (must be eaten)	NOTES
4 oz. orange, grapefruit, *or* tomato juice, *or* 1 orange, *or* ½ grapefruit	May use another fruit, but then one fruit during day must be citrus. Juices must be unsweetened.
AND	
1 egg (made without fat)	
OR	
2 oz. cottage cheese *or* 1 oz. farmer cheese	Use diet cottage cheese if available.
OR	

DIET PLAN 2 (cont.)

¾ oz. hard cheese

OR

2 oz. fish (1 oz. if smoked)

AND

1 slice of *thinly* sliced bread

No butter or margarine!

OR

½ cup of cooked cereal

OR

½ oz. of dry cereal

(with milk from allowance)

Dry cereals must be unsugared. If desired, may have 1 oz. of dry cereal, but give up egg or cheese.

AND

Beverage: tea *or* coffee *or* milk from allowance if desired

Never use milk, cream, or sugar; lemon may be used.

MID-MORNING (if desired—not required)

Tea, coffee, *or* bouillon

In any amount.

LUNCH (do not skip lunch)

Clear soup (any amount) *or* 4 oz. tomato juice if desired (these are optional items)

Soup may be hot or cold, but clear enough to see through.

AND

4 oz. cottage cheese

Preferably diet cottage cheese, but do not worry if it is not.

OR

1 oz. hard cheese

OR

2 eggs

Avoid eating more than 4 eggs per week.

OR

2 oz. meat, fish, shellfish, *or* poultry

Avoid any fish canned in oil.

AND

All the raw vegetable salad you wish—NO LIMIT!

But avoid raw peas.

AND

1 slice of bread

If available, use thinly sliced bread.

OR

½ cup of a cooked vegetable

AND

Beverage

DIET PLAN 2 (cont.)

MID-AFTERNOON (optional)	
Tea, coffee, bouillon, *or* milk from allowance	If still hungry, you may eat raw vegetables freely, and drink a diet soda.
AND	
1 fruit *or* 2 oz. cottage cheese *or* ¾ oz. of hard cheese	
DINNER	
Clear soup *or* 4 oz. tomato juice	
AND	
3 to 4 oz. meat, fish, *or* poultry	Use fish and poultry mostly.
AND	
1 or 2 portions of cooked vegetables, each a ½-cup serving	Never exceed ½ cup per portion; never have a full cup of one vegetable.
AND	
All the raw vegetable salad you desire	Use lemon, vinegar, or some dietetic dressings; never use oil.
AND	
Dessert (not required): 1 fruit *or* ¾ oz. of hard cheese *or* 1 portion dietetic gelatin	
AND	
Beverage	
EVENING (if desired)	
Tea, coffee, *or* milk from allowance	
AND	
1 fruit *or* ¾ oz. hard cheese *or* ¾ oz. of dry cereal with milk from allowance	Measure cereal carefully.

No butter, margarine, oil, mayonnaise, sour or sweet cream, or regular salad dressings

No sugar, honey, jelly, jam, or diet jelly

MILK:

You should have at least one 8-oz. glass of skimmed milk daily: You may have up to two glasses daily.

DIET PLAN 2 (cont.)

ICE CREAM:

You may have 4 oz. (liquid-volume measurement, not weight!) of ice cream or ice milk, three or four times a week in place of a dessert or between-meal snack eaten at the time you are giving up the fruit or cheese. In addition, you must give up a glass of milk for the day. Ice milk is not required, but is preferable to ice cream.

MEAT:

Beef, lamb, and pork (very lean cuts only) are restricted to a maximum of three lunches *and* three dinners per week.

If you miss a food item, you may not make up for it by having it later in the day or at another meal. If you have any doubts, *do not eat it!*

DIET PLAN 3

BREAKFAST (must be eaten)	NOTES
4 oz. orange, grapefruit, *or* tomato juice, *or* 1 orange, *or* ½ grapefruit	May use another fruit, but then one fruit during day must be citrus. Juices must be unsweetened.
AND	
1 egg (made without fat)	
OR	
2 oz. cottage cheese *or* 1 oz. farmer cheese	Use diet cottage cheese if available.
OR	
¾ oz. hard cheese	
OR	
2 oz. fish (1 oz. if smoked)	
AND	
1 slice of *thinly* sliced bread	*No* butter or margarine!
OR	
½ cup of cooked cereal OR ½ oz. of dry cereal } with milk from allowance	Dry cereals must be unsugared. If desired, may have 1 oz. of dry cereal, but give up egg or cheese.
AND	
Beverage: tea *or* coffee *or* milk from allowance if desired	Never use milk, cream, or sugar; lemon may be used.

DIET PLAN 3 (cont.)

MID-MORNING (optional)	
Tea, coffee, *or* bouillon	In any amount.
LUNCH (do not skip lunch)	
Clear soup (any amount) *or* 4 oz. tomato juice (optional)	Soup may be hot or cold, but clear enough to see through.
AND	
4 to 6 oz. cottage cheese	Preferably diet cottage cheese, but do not worry if it is not.
OR	
1½ oz. hard cheese	
OR	
2 eggs	Avoid eating more than 4 eggs per week.
OR	
Up to 3 oz. meat, fish, shellfish, *or* poultry	Avoid any fish canned in oil.
AND	
All the raw vegetable salad you wish—NO LIMIT!	But avoid raw peas.
AND	
1 slice of bread	If available, use thinly sliced bread.
OR	
½ cup of a cooked vegetable	
AND	
Beverage	
MID-AFTERNOON (optional)	
Tea, coffee, bouillon, *or* milk from allowance	If still hungry, you may eat raw vegetables freely, and drink a diet soda.
AND	
1 fruit *or* 2 oz. cottage cheese *or* ¾ oz. of hard cheese	
DINNER	
Clear soup *or* 4 oz. tomato juice	
AND	
4 to 6 oz. meat, fish, *or* poultry	Use fish and poultry mostly.
AND	

DIET PLAN 3 (cont.)

1 or 2 portions of cooked vegetables, each a ½-cup serving	Never exceed ½ cup per portion; never have a full cup of one vegetable.
AND	
All the raw vegetable salad you desire	Use lemon, vinegar, or some dietetic dressings; never use oil.
AND	
Dessert (not required): 1 fruit *or* ¾ oz. of hard cheese or 1 portion dietetic gelatin	
AND	
Beverage	
EVENING (if desired)	
Tea, coffee, *or* milk from allowance	
AND	
1 fruit *or* ¾ oz. hard cheese *or* ¾ oz. of dry cereal with milk from allowance	Measure cereal carefully.

No butter, margarine, oil, mayonnaise, sour or sweet cream, or regular salad dressings

No sugar, honey, jelly, jam, or diet jelly

MILK:

You should have at least one 8-oz. glass of skimmed milk daily; you may have up to two glasses daily.

ICE CREAM:

You may have 4 oz. (liquid-volume measurement, not weight!) of ice cream or ice milk, three or four times a week, in place of a dessert or between-meal snack eaten at the time you are giving up the fruit or cheese. In addition, you must give up a glass of milk for the day. Ice milk is not required, but is preferable to ice cream.

MEAT:

Beef, lamb, and pork (very lean cuts only) are restricted to a maximum of three lunches *and* three dinners per week.

If you miss a food item, you may not make up for it by having it later in the day or at another meal. If you have any doubts, ***do not eat it!***

DIET PLAN 3A

BREAKFAST (must be eaten)	NOTES
4 oz. orange, grapefruit, *or* tomato juice, *or* 1 orange, *or* ½ grapefruit	May use another fruit, but then one fruit during day must be citrus. Juices must be unsweetened.
AND	
1 egg (made without fat)	
OR	
2 oz. cottage cheese *or* 1 oz. farmer cheese	Use diet cottage cheese if available.
OR	
¾ oz. hard cheese	
OR	
2 oz. fish (1 oz. if smoked)	
AND	
1 slice of *thinly* sliced bread	*No* butter or margarine!
OR	
½ cup of cooked cereal OR ½ oz. of dry cereal } with milk from allowance	Dry cereals must be unsugared. If desired, may have 1 oz. of dry cereal, but give up egg or cheese.
AND	
Beverage: tea *or* coffee *or* milk from allowance if desired	Never use milk, cream, or sugar; lemon may be used.
MID-MORNING (if desired—not required)	
Tea, coffee, or bouillon	In any amount.
LUNCH (do not skip lunch)	
Clear soup (any amount) *or* 4 oz. tomato juice if desired (these are optional items)	Soup may be hot or cold, but clear enough to see through.
AND	
4 to 6 oz. cottage cheese	Preferably diet cottage cheese, but do not worry if it is not.
OR	
1½ oz. hard cheese	
OR	
2 eggs	Avoid eating more than 4 eggs per week.
OR	
Up to 3 oz. meat, fish, shellfish, *or* poultry	Avoid any fish canned in oil.
AND	

DIET PLAN 3A (cont.)

All the raw vegetable salad you wish—NO LIMIT!

But avoid raw peas.

AND

1 slice of bread

OR

½ cup of a cooked vegetable

If available, use thinly sliced bread.

AND

Dessert: 1 fruit

AND

Beverage

MID-AFTERNOON (if desired—not required)

Tea, coffee, bouillon, *or* milk from allowance

If still hungry, you may eat raw vegetables freely, and drink a diet soda.

AND

1 fruit *or* 2 oz. cottage cheese *or* ¾ oz. of hard cheese

DINNER

Clear soup *or* 4 oz. tomato juice

AND

4 to 6 oz. meat, fish, *or* poultry

Use fish and poultry mostly.

AND

1 or 2 portions of cooked vegetables, each a ½-cup serving

Never exceed ½ cup per portion; never have a full cup of one vegetable.

AND

All the raw vegetable salad you desire

Use lemon, vinegar, or some dietetic dressings; never use oil.

AND

Dessert (not required): 1 fruit *or* ¾ oz. of hard cheese or 1 portion dietetic gelatin

AND

Beverage

DIET PLAN 3A (cont.)

EVENING (if desired)

Tea, coffee, *or* milk from allowance

AND

1 fruit *or* ¾ oz. hard cheese *or* ¾ oz. of dry cereal with milk from allowance

Measure cereal carefully.

No butter, margarine, oil, mayonnaise, sour or sweet cream, or regular salad dressings

No sugar, honey, jelly, jam, or diet jelly

MILK:

You should have at least one 8-oz. glass of skimmed milk daily; you may have up to two glasses daily.

ICE CREAM:

You may have 4 oz. (liquid-volume measurement, not weight!) of ice cream or ice milk, three or four times a week, in place of a dessert or between-meal snack eaten at the time you are giving up the fruit or cheese. In addition, you must give up a glass of milk for the day. Ice milk is not required, but is preferable to ice cream.

MEAT:

Beef, lamb, and pork (very lean cuts only) are restricted to a maximum of three lunches *and* three dinners per week.

If you miss a food item, you may not make up for it by having it later in the day or at another meal. If you have any doubts, *do not eat it!*

DIET PLAN 3B

BREAKFAST (must be eaten)

4 oz. orange, grapefruit, *or* tomato juice, *or* 1 orange, *or* ½ grapefruit

AND

1 egg (made without fat)

OR

NOTES

May use another fruit, but then one fruit during day must be citrus. Juices must be unsweetened.

DIET PLAN 3B (cont.)

2 oz. cottage cheese *or* 1 oz. farmer cheese OR ¾ oz. hard cheese OR 2 oz. fish (1 oz. if smoked)	Use diet cottage cheese, if available.
AND	
1 slice of *thinly* sliced bread	*No* butter or margarine!
OR	
½ cup of cooked cereal OR ½ oz. of dry cereal } with milk from allowance	Dry cereals must be unsugared. If desired, may have 1 oz. of dry cereal, but give up egg or cheese.
AND	
Beverage: tea *or* coffee *or* milk from allowance if desired	Never use milk, cream, or sugar; lemon may be used.
MID-MORNING (if desired—not required)	
Tea, coffee, *or* bouillon	In any amount.
LUNCH (do not skip lunch) quired)	
Clear soup (any amount) *or* 4 oz. tomato juice if desired (these are optional items)	Soup may be hot or cold, but clear enough to see through.
AND	
4 to 6 oz. cottage cheese	Preferably diet cottage cheese, but do not worry if it is not.
OR	
1½ oz. hard cheese	
OR	
2 eggs	Avoid eating more than 4 eggs per week.
OR	
Up to 3 oz. meat, fish, shellfish, *or* poultry	Avoid any fish canned in oil.
AND	
All the raw vegetable salad you wish—NO LIMIT!	But avoid raw peas.
AND	

DIET PLAN 3B (cont.)

2 slices of bread OR 1 cup of a cooked vegetable	If available, use thinly sliced bread.
AND	
Beverage	
MID-AFTERNOON (if desired—not required)	
Tea, coffee, bouillon, *or* milk from allowance	If still hungry, you may eat raw vegetables freely, and drink a diet soda.
AND	
1 fruit *or* 2 oz. cottage cheese *or* ¾ oz. of hard cheese	
DINNER	
Clear soup *or* 4 oz. tomato juice	
AND	
4 to 6 oz. meat, fish, *or* poultry	Use fish and poultry mostly.
AND	
1 or 2 portions of cooked vegetables, each a ½-cup serving	Never exceed ½ cup per portion; never have a full cup of 1 vegetable.
AND	
All the raw vegetable salad you desire	Use lemon, vinegar, or some dietetic dressings; never use oil.
AND	
Dessert (not required): 1 fruit *or* ¾ oz. of hard cheese *or* 1 portion dietetic gelatin	
AND	
Beverage	
EVENING (if desired)	
Tea, coffee, *or* milk from allowance	
AND	
1 fruit *or* ¾ oz. hard cheese *or* ¾ oz. of dry cereal with milk from allowance	Measure cereal carefully.

DIET PLAN 3B (cont.)

No butter, margarine, oil, mayonnaise, sour or sweet cream, or regular salad dressings

No sugar, honey, jelly, jam, or diet jelly

MILK:

You should have at least one 8-oz. glass of skimmed milk daily; you may have up to two glasses daily.

ICE CREAM:

You may have 4 oz. (liquid-volume measurement, not weight!) of ice cream or ice milk, three or four times a week, in place of a dessert or between-meal snack eaten at the time you are giving up the fruit or cheese. In addition, you must give up a glass of milk for the day. Ice milk is not required, but is preferable to ice cream.

MEAT:

Beef, lamb, and pork (very lean cuts only) are restricted to a maximum of three lunches *and* three dinners per week.

If you miss a food item, you may not make up for it by having it later in the day or at another meal. If you have any doubts, *do not eat it!*

DIET PLAN 3C

BREAKFAST (must be eaten)	NOTES
4 oz. orange, grapefruit, *or* tomato juice, *or* 1 orange, *or* ½ grapefruit	May use another fruit, but then one fruit during day must be citrus. Juices must be unsweetened.
AND	
1 egg (made without fat)	
OR	
2 oz. cottage cheese *or* 1 oz. farmer cheese	Use diet cottage cheese if available.
OR	
¾ oz. hard cheese	
OR	
2 oz. fish (1 oz. if smoked)	
AND	
1 slice of *thinly* sliced bread	*No* butter or margarine!
OR	

DIET PLAN 3C (cont.)

½ cup of cooked cereal OR ½ oz. of dry cereal } with milk from allowance	Dry cereals must be unsugared. If desired, may have 1 oz. of dry cereal, but give up egg or cheese.
AND	
Beverage: tea or coffee or milk from allowance if desired	Never use milk, cream, or sugar; lemon may be used.
MID-MORNING (if desired—not required)	
Tea, coffee, *or* bouillon	In any amount.
LUNCH (do not skip lunch)	
Clear soup (any amount) *or* 4 oz. tomato juice if desired (these are optional items)	Soup may be hot or cold, but clear enough to see through.
AND	
4 to 6 oz. cottage cheese	Preferably diet cottage cheese, but do not worry if it is not.
OR	
1½ oz. hard cheese	
OR	
2 eggs	Avoid eating more than 4 eggs per week.
OR	
Up to 3 oz. meat, fish, shellfish, *or* poultry	Avoid any fish canned in oil.
AND	
All the raw vegetable salad you wish—NO LIMIT!	But avoid raw peas.
AND	
1 slice of bread	If available, use thinly sliced bread.
OR	
½ cup of a cooked vegetable	
AND	
Beverage	
MID-AFTERNOON (if desired—not required)	
Tea, coffee, bouillon, *or* milk from allowance	If still hungry, you may eat raw vegetables freely, and drink a diet soda.
AND	

DIET PLAN 3C (cont.)

1 fruit *or* 2 oz. cottage cheese *or* ¾ oz. of hard cheese

DINNER

Clear soup *or* 4 oz. tomato juice

AND

4 to 6 oz. meat, fish, *or* poultry

Use fish and poultry mostly.

AND

1 or 2 portions of cooked vegetables, each a ½-cup serving

Never exceed a ½ cup per portion; never have a full cup of 1 vegetable.

AND

All the raw vegetable salad you desire

Use lemon, vinegar, or some dietetic dressings; never use oil.

AND

Dessert (not required): 1 fruit *or* ¾ oz. of hard cheese *or* 1 portion dietetic gelatin

AND

Beverage

EVENING (if desired)

Tea, coffee, *or* milk from allowance

AND

1 fruit *or* ¾ oz. hard cheese *or* ¾ oz. of dry cereal with milk from allowance

Measure cereal carefully.

No butter, margarine, oil, mayonnaise, sour or sweet cream, or regular salad dressings

No sugar, honey, jelly, jam, or diet jelly

MILK:

You should have two 8-oz. glasses of skimmed milk daily; you must have at least one glass daily.

ICE CREAM:

You may have 4 oz. (liquid-volume measurement, not weight!) of ice cream or ice milk, three or four times a week, in place of a dessert or between-

DIET PLAN 3D (cont.)

meal snack eaten at the time you are giving up the fruit or cheese. In addition, you must give up a glass of milk for the day. Ice milk is not required, but is preferable to ice cream.

MEAT:

Beef, lamb, and pork (very lean cuts only) are restricted to a maximum of three lunches *and* three dinners per week.

If you miss a food item, you may not make up for it by having it later in the day or at another meal. If you have any doubts, ***do not eat it!***

DIET PLAN 3D

BREAKFAST (must be eaten)	NOTES
4 oz. orange, grapefruit, *or* tomato juice, *or* 1 orange, *or* ½ grapefruit	May use another fruit, but then one fruit during day must be citrus. Juices must be unsweetened.
AND	
1 egg (made without fat)	
OR	
2 oz. cottage cheese *or* 1 oz. farmer cheese	Use diet cottage cheese if available.
OR	
¾ oz. hard cheese	
OR	
2 oz. fish (1 oz. if smoked)	
AND	
1 slice of *thinly* sliced bread	*No* butter or margarine!
OR	
½ cup of cooked cereal OR ½ oz. of dry cereal } with milk from allowance	Dry cereals must be unsugared. If desired, may have 1 oz. of dry cereal, but give up egg or cheese.
AND	
Beverage: tea or coffee or milk from allowance if desired	Never use milk, cream, or sugar; lemon may be used.
MID-MORNING (if desired—not required)	
Tea, coffee, or bouillon	In any amount.

DIET PLAN 3D (cont.)

LUNCH (do not skip lunch)

Clear soup (any amount) *or* 4 oz. tomato juice if desired (these are optional items)	Soup may be hot or cold, but clear enough to see through.
AND	
4 to 6 oz. cottage cheese OR 1½ oz. hard cheese OR	Preferably diet cottage cheese, but do not worry if it is not.
2 eggs OR	Avoid eating more than 4 eggs per week.
Up to 3 oz. meat, fish, shellfish, *or* poultry	Avoid any fish canned in oil.
AND	
All the raw vegetable salad you wish—NO LIMIT!	But avoid raw peas.
AND	
1 or 2 slices of bread* OR ½ to 1 cup of cooked vegetables	If available, use thinly sliced bread.
AND/OR	
Dessert: 1 fruit*	
AND	
Beverage	

MID-AFTERNOON (if desired—not required)

Tea, coffee, bouillon, *or* milk from allowance	If still hungry, you may eat raw vegetables freely, and drink a diet soda.
AND	
1 fruit *or* 2 oz. cottage cheese *or* ¾ oz. of hard cheese	

---

* A choice of 2 slices of bread (closed sandwich) and no dessert, *or* 1 slice of bread (open sandwich) and a dessert.

DIET PLAN 3D (cont.)

DINNER

Clear soup *or* 4 oz. tomato juice	
AND	
4 to 6 oz. meat, fish, *or* poultry	Use fish and poultry mostly.
AND	
1 or 2 portions of cooked vegetables, each a ½ cup	Never exceed ½ cup per portion; never have a full cup of 1 vegetable.
AND	
All the raw vegetable salad you desire	Use lemon, vinegar, or some dietetic dressings; never use oil.
AND	
Dessert (not required): 1 fruit *or* ¾ oz. of hard cheese *or* 1 portion dietetic gelatin	
AND	
Beverage	

EVENING (if desired)

Tea, coffee, *or* milk from allowance	
AND	
1 fruit *or* ¾ oz. hard cheese *or* ¾ oz. of dry cereal with milk from allowance	Measure cereal carefully.

No butter, margarine, oil, mayonnaise, sour or sweet cream, or regular salad dressings

No sugar, honey, jelly, jam, or diet jelly

MILK:

You should have two or three 8-oz. glasses of skimmed milk daily; you must have at least 1 glass daily.

ICE CREAM:

You may have 4 oz. (liquid-volume measurement, not weight!) of ice cream or ice milk, three or four times a week, in place of a dessert or between-meal snack eaten at the time you are giving up the fruit or cheese. In addition, you must give up a glass of milk for the day. Ice milk is not required, but is preferable to ice cream.

DIET PLAN 3D (cont.)

MEAT:

Beef, lamb, and pork (very lean cuts only) are restricted to a maximum of three lunches *and* three dinners per week.

If you miss a food item, you may not make up for it by having it later in the day or at another meal. If you have any doubts, ***do not eat it!***

DIET PLAN 3E

BREAKFAST (must be eaten)	NOTES
4 oz. orange, grapefruit, *or* tomato juice, *or* 1 orange, *or* ½ grapefruit	May use another fruit, but then one fruit during day must be citrus. Juices must be unsweetened.
AND	
1 egg (made without fat)	
OR	
2 oz. cottage cheese *or* 1 oz. farmer cheese	Use diet cottage cheese if available.
OR	
¾ oz. hard cheese	
OR	
2 oz. fish (1 oz. if smoked)	
AND	
1 slice of *thinly* sliced bread	*No* butter or margarine!
OR	
½ cup of cooked cereal OR ½ oz. of dry cereal } with milk from allowance	Dry cereals must be unsugared. If desired, may have 1 oz. of dry cereal, but give up egg or cheese.
AND	
Beverage: milk from allowance if desired	
LUNCH (do not skip lunch)	
Clear soup (any amount) *or* 4 oz. tomato juice if desired (these are optional items)	Soup may be hot or cold, but clear enough to see through.
AND	
4 to 6 oz. cottage cheese	Preferably diet cottage cheese, but do not worry if it is not.
OR	
1½ oz. hard cheese	
OR	

DIET PLAN 3E (cont.)

2 eggs OR Up to 3 oz. meat, fish, shellfish, *or* poultry	Avoid eating more than 4 eggs per week. Avoid any fish canned in oil.
AND	
All the raw vegetable salad you wish—NO LIMIT!	But avoid raw peas.
AND	
2 slices of bread OR 1 cup of cooked vegetables	May have 1 slice of bread *and* ½ cup of cooked vegetables.
AND	
Dessert: 1 fruit	
AND	
Beverage	
MID-AFTERNOON (if desired—not required)	
Milk from allowance	You may eat raw vegetables freely, and drink a diet soda.
AND	
1 fruit	
DINNER	
Clear soup *or* 4 oz. tomato juice	
AND	
4 to 6 oz. meat, fish, *or* poultry	Use fish and poultry mostly.
AND	
1 or 2 portions of cooked vegetables, each a ½-cup serving	Never exceed ½ cup per portion; never have a full cup of 1 vegetable
AND	
All the raw vegetable salad you desire	Use lemon, vinegar, or some dietetic dressings; never use oil.
AND	

DIET PLAN 3E (cont.)

Dessert (not required): 1 fruit *or* ¾ oz. of hard cheese or 1 portion dietetic gelatin

AND

Beverage

EVENING (optional)

Milk from allowance

AND

1 fruit

No butter, margarine, oil, mayonnaise, sour or sweet cream, or regular salad dressings

No sugar, honey, jelly, jam, or diet jelly

You may have 1 starch vegetable once a week (potato, rice, noodles, spaghetti, etc.) *and* 2 cookies once a week.

MILK:

You should have three 8-oz. glasses of skimmed milk daily, and must have at least two glasses.

ICE CREAM:

You may have 4 oz. (liquid-volume measurement, not weight!) of ice cream or ice milk, in place of a dessert or between-meal snack eaten at the time you are giving up the fruit or cheese. In addition, you must give up a glass of milk for the day. Ice milk is not required, but is preferable to ice cream.

MEAT:

Beef, lamb and pork (very lean cuts only) are restricted to a maximum of three lunches *and* three dinners per week.

If you miss a food item, you may not make up for it by having it later in the day or at another meal. If you have any doubts, *do not eat it!*

DIET PLAN 4

BREAKFAST (must be eaten)

4 oz. orange, grapefruit, *or* tomato juice, *or* 1 orange, *or* ½ grapefruit

AND

NOTES

May use another fruit, but then one fruit during day must be citrus. Juices must be unsweetened.

DIET PLAN 4 (cont.)

1 egg (made without fat)

OR

2 oz. cottage cheese *or* 1 oz. farmer cheese — Use diet cottage cheese if available.

OR

¾ oz. hard cheese

OR

2 oz. fish (1 oz. if smoked)

AND

1 slice of *thinly* sliced bread — *No* butter or margarine!

OR

½ cup of cooked cereal OR ½ oz. of dry cereal — with milk from allowance — Dry cereals must be unsugared. If desired, may have 1 oz. of dry cereal, but give up egg or cheese.

AND

Beverage: tea *or* coffee *or* milk from allowance if desired — Never use milk, cream, or sugar; lemon may be used.

MID-MORNING (if desired—not required)

Tea, coffee, *or* bouillon — In any amount.

LUNCH (do not skip lunch)

Clear soup (any amount) *or* 4 oz. tomato juice if desired (these are optional items) — Soup may be hot or cold, but clear enough to see through.

AND

6 to 8 oz. cottage cheese — Preferably diet cottage cheese, but do not worry if it is not.

OR

2 oz. hard cheese

OR

2 eggs — Avoid eating more than 4 eggs per week.

OR

Up to 4 oz. meat, fish, shellfish, *or* poultry — Avoid any fish canned in oil.

AND

All the raw vegetable salad you wish—NO LIMIT! — But avoid raw peas.

AND

DIET PLAN 4 (cont.)

2 slices of bread OR 1 cup of cooked vegetables	May have one slice of bread *and* ½ cup of cooked vegetables.
AND	
Dessert (not required): 1 fruit	
AND	
Beverage	
MID-AFTERNOON (if desired—not required)	
Tea, coffee, bouillon, *or* milk from allowance	If still hungry, you may eat raw vegetables freely, and drink a diet soda.
AND	
1 fruit *or* 2 oz. cottage cheese *or* ¾ oz. of hard cheese	
DINNER	
Clear soup *or* 4 oz. tomato juice	
AND	
6 to 8 oz. meat, fish, *or* poultry	Use fish and poultry mostly.
AND	
1 or 2 portions of cooked vegetables, each a ½-cup serving	Never exceed ½ cup per portion; never have a full cup of 1 vegetable.
AND	
All the raw vegetable salad you desire	Use lemon, vinegar, or some dietetic dressings; never use oil.
AND	
Dessert (not required): 1 fruit *or* ¾ oz. of hard cheese *or* 1 portion dietetic gelatin	
AND	
Beverage	
EVENING (if desired)	
Tea, coffee, *or* milk from allowance	
AND	

DIET PLAN 4 (cont.)

1 fruit *or* ¾ oz. hard cheese *or* ¾ oz. of dry cereal with milk from allowance	Measure cereal carefully.

No butter, margarine, oil, mayonnaise, sour or sweet cream, or regular salad dressings

No sugar, honey, jelly, jam, or diet jelly

MILK:

You should have at least one 8-oz. glass of skimmed milk daily; you may have up to two glasses daily.

ICE CREAM:

You may have 4 oz. (liquid-volume measurement, not weight!) of ice cream or ice milk, three or four times a week in place of a dessert or between-meal snack eaten at the time you are giving up the fruit or cheese. In addition, you must give up a glass of milk for the day. Ice milk is not required, but is preferable to ice cream.

MEAT:

Beef, lamb, and pork (very lean cuts only) are restricted to a maximum of three lunches *and* three dinners per week.

If you miss a food item, you may not make up for it by having it later in the day or at another meal. If you have any doubts, *do not eat it!*

DIET PLAN 4A

BREAKFAST (must be eaten)	NOTES
4 oz. orange, grapefruit, *or* tomato juice, *or* 1 orange, *or* ½ grapefruit	May use another fruit, but then one fruit during day must be citrus. Juices must be unsweetened.
AND	
1 or 2 eggs (made without fat)	
OR	
2 to 4 oz. cottage cheese *or* 1 to 2 oz. farmer cheese	Use diet cottage cheese if available.
OR	
1½ oz. hard cheese	
OR	
2 to 3 oz. fish (1 to 1½ oz. if smoked)	
AND	

DIET PLAN 4A (cont.)

1 or 2 slices of *thinly* sliced bread

No butter or margarine!

OR

½ to 1 cup of cooked cereal
OR
½ to 1 oz. of dry cereal
} with milk from allowance

Dry cereals must be unsugared. If desired, may have 1 oz. of dry cereal, but give up egg or cheese.

AND

Beverage: tea or coffee or milk from allowance if desired

Never use milk, cream, or sugar; lemon may be used.

MID-MORNING (if desired—not required)

Tea, coffee, *or* bouillon

In any amount.

LUNCH (do not skip lunch)

Clear soup (any amount) *or* 4 oz. tomato juice if desired (these are optional items)

Soup may be hot or cold, but clear enough to see through.

AND

6 to 8 oz. cottage cheese

Preferably diet cottage cheese, but do not worry if it is not.

OR

2 oz. hard cheese

OR

2 eggs

Avoid eating more than 4 eggs per week.

OR

Up to 4 oz. meat, fish, shellfish, *or* poultry

Avoid any fish canned in oil.

AND

All the raw vegetable salad you wish—NO LIMIT!

But avoid raw peas.

AND

2 slices of bread

OR

1 cup of cooked vegetables

May have one slice of bread *and* ½ cup of cooked vegetables.

AND

Dessert (not required): 1 fruit

AND

Beverage

DIET PLAN 4A (cont.)

MID-AFTERNOON (if desired—not required)	
Tea, coffee, bouillon, *or* milk from allowance	If still hungry, you may eat raw vegetables freely, and drink a diet soda.
AND	
1 fruit *or* 2 oz. cottage cheese *or* ¾ oz. of hard cheese	
DINNER	
Clear soup *or* 4 oz. tomato juice	
AND	
6 to 8 oz. meat, fish, *or* poultry	Use fish and poultry mostly.
AND	
1 or 2 portions of cooked vegetables, each a ½-cup serving	Never exceed ½ cup per portion; never have a full cup of 1 vegetable.
AND	
All the raw vegetable salad you desire	Use lemon, vinegar, or some dietetic dressings; never use oil.
AND	
Dessert (not required): 1 fruit *or* ¾ oz. of hard cheese or 1 portion dietetic gelatin	
AND	
Beverage	
EVENING (if desired)	
Tea, coffee, *or* milk from allowance	
AND	
1 fruit *or* ¾ oz. hard cheese *or* ¾ oz. of dry cereal with milk from allowance	Measure cereal carefully.

No butter, margarine, oil, mayonnaise, sour or sweet cream, or regular salad dressings

No sugar, honey, jelly, jam, or diet jelly

DIET PLAN 4A (cont.)

MILK:

You should have at least one 8-oz. glass of skimmed milk daily; you may have up to two glasses daily.

ICE CREAM:

You may have 4 oz. (liquid-volume measurement, not weight!) of ice cream or ice milk, three or four times a week, in place of a dessert or between-meal snack eaten at the time you are giving up the fruit or cheese. In addition, you must give up a glass of milk for the day. Ice milk is not required, but is preferable to ice cream.

MEAT:

Beef, lamb, and pork (very lean cuts only) are restricted to a maximum of three lunches *and* three dinners per week.

If you miss a food item, you may not make up for it by having it later in the day or at another meal. If you have any doubts, *do not eat it!*

DIET PLAN 4B

BREAKFAST (must be eaten)	NOTES
4 oz. orange, grapefruit, *or* tomato juice, *or* 1 orange, *or* ½ grapefruit	May use another fruit, but then one fruit during day must be citrus. Juices must be unsweetened.
AND	
1 egg (made without fat)	
OR	
2 oz. cottage cheese *or* 1 oz. farmer cheese	Use diet cottage cheese if available.
OR	
¾ oz. hard cheese	
OR	
2 oz. fish (1 oz. if smoked)	
AND	
1 slice of *thinly* sliced bread	*No* butter or margarine!
OR	
½ cup of cooked cereal OR ½ oz. of dry cereal } with milk from allowance	Dry cereals must be unsugared. If desired, may have 1 oz. of dry cereal, but give up egg or cheese.
AND	
Beverage: tea or coffee or milk from allowance if desired	Never use milk, cream, or sugar; lemon may be used.

DIET PLAN 4B (cont.)

MID-MORNING (if desired—not required)	
Tea, coffee, or bouillon	In any amount.
LUNCH (do not skip lunch)	
Clear soup (any amount) *or* 4 oz. tomato juice if desired (these are optional items)	Soup may be hot or cold, but clear enough to see through.
AND	
6 to 8 oz. cottage cheese	Preferably diet cottage cheese, but do not worry if it is not.
OR	
2 oz. hard cheese	
OR	
2 eggs	Avoid eating more than 4 eggs per week.
Up to 4 oz. meat, fish, shellfish, *or* poultry	Avoid any fish canned in oil.
AND	
All the raw vegetable salad you wish—NO LIMIT!	But avoid raw peas.
AND	
2 slices of bread	May have 1 slice of bread *and* ½ cup of cooked vegetables.
OR	
1 cup of cooked vegetables	
AND	
Dessert: 1 fruit	
AND	
Beverage	
MID-AFTERNOON (if desired—not required)	
Tea, coffee, bouillon, *or* milk from allowance	If still hungry, you may eat raw vegetables freely, and drink a diet soda.
AND	
1 fruit *or* 2 oz. cottage cheese *or* ¾ oz. of hard cheese	

DIET PLAN 4B (cont.)

DINNER

Clear soup *or* 4 oz. tomato juice

AND

Girls: 4 to 6 oz. meat, fish, or poultry
Boys: 4 to 8 oz. meat, fish, or poultry

Use fish and poultry mostly.

AND

1 or 2 portions of cooked vegetables, each a ½-cup serving

Never exceed ½ cup per portion; never have a full cup of 1 vegetable.

AND

All the raw vegetable salad you desire

Use lemon, vinegar, or some dietetic dressings; never use oil.

AND

Dessert (optional): 1 fruit *or* ¾ oz. of hard cheese *or* 1 portion dietetic gelatin

AND

Beverage

EVENING (if desired)

Tea, coffee, *or* milk from allowance

AND

1 fruit *or* ¾ oz. hard cheese

No butter, margarine, oil, mayonnaise, sour or sweet cream, or regular salad dressings

No sugar, honey, jelly, jam, or diet jelly

MILK:

Boys should have three 8-oz. glasses of skimmed milk daily, and must have at least two glasses daily.

Girls should have two or three 8-oz. glasses of skimmed milk daily, and must have at least one glass daily.

ICE CREAM:

You may have 4 oz. (liquid-volume measurement, not weight!) of ice cream or ice milk, three or four times a week, in place of a dessert or between-meal snack eaten at the time you are giving up the fruit or cheese. In addition, you must give up a glass of milk for the day. Ice milk is not required, but is preferable to ice cream.

DIET PLAN 4B (cont.)

MEAT:

Beef, lamb, and pork (very lean cuts only) are restricted to a maximum of three lunches *and* three dinners per week.

If you miss a food item, you may not make up for it by having it later in the day or at another meal. If you have any doubts, *do not eat it!*

DIET PLAN 4C

BREAKFAST (must be eaten)	NOTES
4 oz. orange, grapefruit, *or* tomato juice, *or* 1 orange, *or* ½ grapefruit	May use another fruit, but then one fruit during day must be citrus. Juices must be unsweetened.
AND	
1 or 2 eggs (made without fat)	
OR	
2 to 4 oz. cottage cheese *or* 1 to 2 oz. farmer cheese	Use diet cottage cheese if available.
OR	
¾ to 1½ oz. hard cheese	
OR	
2 to 3 oz. fish (1 to 1½ oz. if smoked)	
AND	
1 or 2 slices of *thinly* sliced bread	*No* butter or margarine!
OR	
½ to 1 cup of cooked cereal OR ½ to 1 oz. of dry cereal } with milk from allowance	Dry cereals must be unsugared.
AND	
Beverage: tea or coffee or milk from allowance if desired	Never use milk, cream, or sugar; lemon may be used.
MID-MORNING (optional)	
Tea, coffee, *or* bouillon	In any amount.
LUNCH (do not skip lunch)	
Clear soup (any amount) *or* 4 oz. tomato juice if desired (these are optional items)	Soup may be hot or cold, but clear enough to see through.
AND	

DIET PLAN 4C (cont.)

6 to 8 oz. cottage cheese	Preferably diet cottage cheese, but do not worry if it is not.
OR	
2 oz. hard cheese	
OR	
2 eggs	Avoid eating more than 4 eggs per week.
OR	
Up to 4 oz. meat, fish, shellfish, *or* poultry	Avoid any fish canned in oil.
AND	
All the raw vegetable salad you wish—NO LIMIT!	But avoid raw peas.
AND	
2 slices of bread	May have 1 slice of bread *and* ½ cup of cooked vegetables.
OR	
1 cup of cooked vegetables	
AND	
Dessert: 1 fruit	
AND	
Beverage	
MID-AFTERNOON (if desired—not required)	
Tea, coffee, bouillon, *or* milk from allowance	If still hungry, you may eat raw vegetables freely, and drink a diet soda.
AND	
1 fruit *and* 2 oz. cottage cheese *or* ¾ oz. of hard cheese, *or* 2 fruits and no cheese	
DINNER	
Clear soup *or* 4 oz. tomato juice	
AND	
6 to 8 oz. meat, fish, *or* poultry	Use fish and poultry mostly.
AND	
1 or 2 portions of cooked vegetables, each a ½-cup serving	Never exceed ½ cup per portion; never have a full cup of 1 vegetable.
AND	

DIET PLAN 4C (cont.)

All the raw vegetable salad you desire

Use lemon, vinegar, or some dietetic dressings; never use oil.

AND

Dessert (not required): 1 fruit *or* ¾ oz. of hard cheese *or* 1 portion dietetic gelatin

AND

Beverage

EVENING (if desired)

Tea, coffee, *or* milk from allowance

AND

1 fruit *or* ¾ oz. hard cheese *or* ¾ oz. of dry cereal with milk from allowance

Measure cereal carefully.

No butter, margarine, oil, mayonnaise, sour or sweet cream, or regular salad dressings

No sugar, honey, jelly, jam, or diet jelly

MILK:

You should have three 8-oz. glasses of skimmed milk daily, and must have at least two glasses daily.

ICE CREAM:

You may have 4 oz. (liquid-volume measurement, not weight!) of ice cream or ice milk, three or four times a week, in place of a dessert or between-meal snack eaten at the time you are giving up the fruit or cheese. In addition, you must give up a glass of milk for the day. Ice milk is not required, but is preferable to ice cream.

MEAT:

Beef, lamb, and pork (very lean cuts only) are restricted to a maximum of three lunches *and* three dinners per week.

If you miss a food item, you may not make up for it by having it later in the day or at another meal. If you have any doubts, *do not eat it!*

DIET PLAN 5

BREAKFAST (must be eaten)	NOTES
4 oz. orange, grapefruit, *or* tomato juice, *or* 1 orange, *or* ½ grapefruit	May use another fruit, but then one fruit during day must be citrus. Juices must be unsweetened.
AND	
1 egg (made without fat)	
OR	
2 oz. cottage cheese *or* 1 oz. farmer cheese	Use diet cottage cheese if available.
OR	
¾ oz. hard cheese	
OR	
2 oz. fish (1 oz. if smoked)	
AND	
1 slice of *thinly* sliced bread	*No* butter or margarine!
OR	
½ cup of cooked cereal OR ½ oz. of dry cereal } with milk from allowance	Dry cereals must be unsugared. If desired, may have 1 oz. of dry cereal, but give up egg or cheese.
AND	
Beverage: tea *or* coffee *or* milk from allowance if desired	Never use milk, cream, or sugar; lemon may be used.
MID-MORNING (if desired—not required)	
Tea, coffee, *or* bouillon	In any amount.
LUNCH (do not skip lunch)	
Clear soup (any amount) *or* 4 oz. tomato juice if desired (these are optional items)	Soup may be hot or cold, but clear enough to see through.
AND	
8 to 12 oz. cottage cheese	Preferably diet cottage cheese, but do not worry if it is not.
OR	
2 to 4 oz. hard cheese	
OR	
2 eggs	Avoid eating more than 4 eggs per week.
OR	
Up to 4 to 6 oz. meat, fish, shellfish, *or* poultry	Avoid any fish canned in oil.
AND	

DIET PLAN 5 (cont.)

All the raw vegetable salad you wish—NO LIMIT!	But avoid raw peas.
AND	
2 to 4 slices of bread OR 1 cup of cooked vegetables	This will provide two sandwiches if desired.
AND	
Dessert: 1 fruit	
AND	
Beverage	
MID-AFTERNOON (if desired—not required)	
Tea, coffee, bouillon, *or* milk from allowance	If still hungry, you may eat raw vegetables freely, and drink a diet soda.
AND	
1 fruit *or* 2 oz. cottage cheese *or* ¾ oz. hard cheese	
DINNER	
Clear soup *or* 4 oz. tomato juice	
AND	
6 to 8 oz. meat, fish, *or* poultry	Use fish and poultry mostly.
AND	
1 or 2 portions of cooked vegetables, each a ½-cup serving	Never exceed ½ cup per portion; never have a full cup of 1 vegetable.
AND	
All the raw vegetable salad you desire	Use lemon, vinegar, or some dietetic dressings; never use oil.
AND	
Dessert (not required): 1 fruit *or* ¾ oz. of hard cheese *or* 1 portion dietetic gelatin	
AND	
Beverage	

DIET PLAN 5 (cont.)

EVENING (if desired)

Tea, coffee, *or* milk from allowance

AND

1 fruit *or* ¾ oz. hard cheese *or* ¾ oz. of dry cereal with milk from allowance

Measure cereal carefully.

OR

If desired, have only one sandwich at lunch (using only half quantities of the main course) and have the other sandwich now instead of at lunch time.

No butter, margarine, oil, mayonnaise, sour or sweet cream, or regular salad dressings

No sugar, honey, jelly, jam, or diet jelly

MILK:

You should have at least one 8-oz. glass of skimmed milk daily; you may have up to two glasses daily.

ICE CREAM:

You may have 4 oz. (liquid-volume measurement, not weight!) of ice cream or ice milk, three or four times a week in place of a dessert or between-meal snack eaten at the time you are giving up the fruit or cheese. In addition, you must give up a glass of milk for the day. Ice milk is not required, but is preferable to ice cream.

MEAT:

Beef, lamb, and pork (very lean cuts only) are restricted to a maximum of three lunches *and* three dinners per week.

If you miss a food item, you may not make up for it by having it later in the day or at another meal. If you have any doubts, *do not eat it!*

DIET PLAN 5A

BREAKFAST (must be eaten)

4 oz. orange, grapefruit, *or* tomato juice, *or* 1 orange, *or* ½ grapefruit

AND

NOTES

May use another fruit, but then one fruit during day must be citrus. Juices must be unsweetened.

DIET PLAN 5A (cont.)

2 eggs (made without fat)	
OR	
4 oz. cottage cheese *or* 2 oz. farmer cheese	Use the cottage cheese if available.
OR	
1½ oz. hard cheese	
OR	
3 oz. fish (1½ oz. if smoked)	
AND	
2 slices of *thinly* sliced bread	*No* butter or margarine!
OR	
1 cup of cooked cereal OR 1 oz. of dry cereal } with milk from allowance	Dry cereals must be unsugared.
AND	
Beverage: tea *or* coffee *or* milk from allowance if desired	Never use milk, cream, or sugar; lemon may be used.
MID-MORNING (if desired—not required)	
Tea, coffee, *or* bouillon	In any amount.
LUNCH (do not skip lunch)	
Clear soup (any amount) *or* 4 oz. tomato juice if desired (these are optional items)	Soup may be hot or cold, but clear enough to see through.
AND	
8 to 12 oz. cottage cheese	Preferably diet cottage cheese, but do not worry if it is not.
OR	
2 to 4 oz. hard cheese	
OR	
2 eggs	Avoid eating more than 4 eggs per week.
OR	
Up to 4 to 6 oz. meat, fish, shellfish, *or* poultry	Avoid any fish canned in oil.
AND	
All the raw vegetable salad you wish—NO LIMIT!	But avoid raw peas.
AND	

DIET PLAN 5A (cont.)

2 to 4 slices of bread

OR

1 cup of cooked vegetables

This will provide two sandwiches if desired.

AND

Dessert: 1 fruit

AND

Beverage

MID-AFTERNOON (if desired—not required)

Tea, coffee, bouillon, *or* milk from allowance

If still hungry, you may eat raw vegetables freely, and drink a diet soda.

AND

1 fruit *and* ¾ oz. of hard cheese, *or* 2 fruits and no cheese

DINNER

Clear soup *or* 4 oz. tomato juice

AND

4 to 6 oz. meat, fish, *or* poultry

Use fish and poultry mostly.

AND

1 or 2 portions of cooked vegetables, each a ½-cup serving

Never exceed ½ cup per portion; never have a full cup of 1 vegetable

AND

1 slice of bread

AND

All the raw vegetable salad you desire

Use lemon, vinegar, or some dietetic dressings; never use oil.

AND

Dessert (not required): 1 fruit *or* ¾ oz. of hard cheese, *or* 1 portion dietetic gelatin

AND

Beverage

DIET PLAN 5A (cont.)

EVENING (if desired)

Tea, coffee, *or* milk from allowance

AND

1 fruit *or* ¾ oz. hard cheese

OR

If desired, have only one sandwich at lunch (using only half quantities of the main course) and have the other sandwich now instead of at lunch time.

No butter, margarine, oil, mayonnaise, sour or sweet cream, or regular salad dressings

No sugar, honey, jelly, jam, or diet jelly

MILK:

You should have three 8-oz. glasses of skimmed milk daily, and must have at least two glasses daily.

ICE CREAM:

You may have 4 oz. (liquid-volume measurement, not weight!) of ice cream or ice milk, three or four times a week, in place of a dessert or between-meal snack eaten at the time you are giving up the fruit or cheese. In addition, you must give up a glass of milk for the day. Ice milk is not required, but is preferable to ice cream.

MEAT:

Beef, lamb, and pork (very lean cuts only) are restricted to a maximum of three lunches *and* three dinners per week.

If you miss a food item, you may not make up for it by having it later in the day or at another meal. If you have any doubts, *do not eat it!*

6

Planning and Timing Your Meals

Meal timing in using the Diet Plans is based on the principle that you have breakfast within 1 hour of arising, and that lunch is approximately 4 hours later. Inasmuch as your blood sugar level is low about 4 hours after eating, and inasmuch as dinner for most people is about 6 hours after lunch, a snack is allowed in the afternoon. For the same reason, a snack is allowed at bedtime.

Now, here are a number of important questions and answers that are very often asked regarding problems connected with meals and timing.

If I am not hungry, may I skip breakfast?

No meal may be skipped, and least of all breakfast. Breakfast is the meal that *starts* a good day of dieting. Many people say that they are not hungry in the morning. They do not want to eat, and, in fact, often say they *cannot* eat. And then they add, "Won't it save calories?" If you want to save calories, give up dinner, the meal that contains the most calories! *The answer to dieting is not how little you eat, but how correctly you eat.* It is the correctness that will give you the ability to stay on the diet, and, most of all, to develop the food habits that will help you to keep the weight off permanently.

When one skips a meal, there is a risk of being too hungry later and, therefore, truly going off the diet and eating more calories than were "saved" by the missed meal.

What is "hidden" hunger?

When one skips breakfast, hunger begins gradually to build up. It is not realized at first, which is why I call it a *hidden* hunger. The traditional pattern of the overweight individual is to eat very little during the first part of the day and then overeat as the day progresses, often gorging himself at night. Then, naturally, he is still stuffed and not hungry early in the morning. This cycle must be broken. One *must* eat breakfast on these diets, and preferably it should be eaten within an hour of arising.

What if I get up too late for breakfast?

Some individuals who stay up very late often get up very late. They would be better off starting their day with breakfast, and simply pushing their other two meals back in time. If you do not stay up extra late, and you arise *after* 11:00 A.M., then, and only then should you skip breakfast. Do not combine breakfast and lunch, but rather, simply add a citrus fruit to your lunch.

Is it ever possible to have a bigger breakfast particularly on Sundays or on vacation?

No. Do not have a bigger breakfast. Just because one has more time to eat does not mean that eating should become a major occupation. This is not a lifetime prohibition, but it is a rigid rule while dieting.

What should I do if lunch is eaten very late and there is a longer period of time between lunch and breakfast than the usual four hours?

Under these circumstances I suggest that you take one fruit at midmorning and skip either the afternoon or the bedtime fruit.

Can lunch and dinner be reversed?

Yes, but make it a total switch, rather than switching part of a meal. There is no objection to eating breakfast on arising, dinner as the midday meal, and lunch as the evening meal.

How do you handle eating if you go to night school after work and come home rather late?

In these circumstances most people are too rushed after work to have a regular dinner and too tired after school to prepare a full dinner. The way to handle this is to divide the dinner into two lunches. Have one lunch just before school starts and the second lunch after school, using a sandwich form of meal if desired. In other words, on night-school days you have breakfast in the morning, lunch at the usual noon hour, a second lunch before you go to class, and the third lunch when you come home.

Have your dinner fruit with the preschool lunch and the bedtime fruit with the after-school lunch. Experience has shown this to be a very workable and satisfactory technique.

What should I do if I wake up about two in the morning and feel the need to eat something?

First of all, of course, try to control the urge. If you cannot, then I suggest that you do the following: Save one of your glasses of skimmed milk for this time. If you do wake up, drink it; if you do not wake up, simply skip it. If this is not enough, keep low-calorie gelatin in the refrigerator. Make this in advance so it is always available, and eat it freely if you awaken during the night. Eating the milk and gelatin should be enough to allow you to go back to sleep.

If a food item is skipped at one meal, may I have it at the following meal?

No. Once an item is gone, it is gone. Meal patterning is the true basis of weight control during maintenance (which means keeping to your correct weight permanently after you have reached it). Learn it as you lose weight. Do not get fooled by the arithmetic of weight reduction.

If I do not have beef or lamb at lunch, may I have these meats more often at dinner?

No. On these diet plans, one must truly adjust to having less beef and lamb. Never exceed three beef–lamb lunches and dinners per week.

Is there any objection to a cold supper?

No, but keep this type of a meal to a minimum. It is important to maintain the dinner form. There is no objection to eating your vegetables, such as beets or asparagus, cold. If you are trapped in unusual circumstances, you may substitute one slice of bread for each ½-cup vegetable portion allowed.

May a food item such as turkey or Wheaties be repeated on consecutive days?

There is no objection to this, but obviously the more variety, the better.

We may now turn from the Diet Plans and the timing of meals to the planning and control of diet meals in terms of the various groups of foods. In the questions and answers in the following chapters, we shall discuss the various foods and customary courses in specific detail, starting with the first course.

7

First Courses

First courses or appetizers are optional in your Diet Plan, but are carefully controlled. If you are in a restaurant, the appetizer can keep you busy so that you are not tempted to eat bread while waiting for your food to be ready. Incidentally, another good trick to help you keep away from the bread while waiting to be served is to order a dish of raw celery and carrots. Most restaurants will serve it on request. But if they serve olives with it, do not eat them.

What first courses (appetizers) are allowed?

There are two basic categories of the first course: soups and juices. The soups may be eaten hot or cold (jellied consommés and madrilene are allowed). The primary rule about soups is that they must be clear—clear enough to see through. This basically limits the soups to consommé, bouillon, or broth. All homemade soups should have all fat skimmed off. This is best done by allowing them to cool off in the refrigerator. The fat will rise to the top, and it then can be easily removed. The broth can then be reheated and served. If anything is floating in the soup, I do not consider it clear. It is not adequate to eat from the top of the soup and leave the noodles or rice at the bottom.

The best juices are tomato juice, V-8, clam juice, or diet cranberry juice. Avoid all other fruit juices because they have more calories than those juices that are allowed.

Is there any objection to instant soups?

No, as long as the instant soups add up to less than 12 calories per serving (most instant soup labels state the number of calories per serving). These may be used as an appetizer or as a free snack between meals.

Can beet soup (borscht) be used?

We do not permit any soups that are not clear enough to see through. If there is a special dietary beet soup available, it must have less than 12 calories per serving to be allowed.

May I have gaspacho soup?

Absolutely not! Gaspacho is not a clear soup and, incidentally, if made properly, it contains oil.

May smoked fish be used as a first course or appetizer?

Following the half-quantity rule explained on page 99, smoked fish may be eaten as an appetizer on condition that you subtract the quantity from the quantity of main course allowed. If your Diet Plan calls for 6 ounces of main course at dinner, you could have 1 ounce of smoked salmon as an appetizer. Since this is equivalent to 2 ounces of nonsmoked fish, your main course would be limited to a 4-ounce portion.

May shrimp be used as an appetizer?

Yes, but the quantity (in ounces) should be deducted from the main-course protein.

Are hors d'oeuvres (antipasto) allowed?

Only if you pick and choose the items in the hors d'oeuvres very carefully (see below). Be particularly careful to avoid any items prepared with oil.

What may I eat for hors d'oeuvres?

The only hors d'oeuvres allowed are raw vegetables, but there are many: carrots, cucumbers, string beans, zucchini, to name a few. If you are at a large, fancy party, and hors d'oeuvres are served garnished with fresh vegetables, do not be afraid to eat the garnishes.

You will recall that there is a general rule never to eat unless you are sitting down. Remembering this rule will help you considerably in controlling the nibbling you are otherwise likely to do at parties. And remember, it is easier not to take the first hors d'oeuvre than it is the second and third!

8

Meats and Fish: High-Quality Proteins for Main Courses

Meals are generally built around the main course. When one is asked what he had for dinner or lunch, the answer is usually a one- or two-word response, simply citing the main course. The main course is the major item, not only for satisfaction, but also in calories. For the vast majority of individuals, *the largest number of calories in any one meal is invariably found in the main course*. Accordingly, the dieter must pay constant attention to these main courses. Calories are best saved by careful attention to main courses.

Many of the questions my patients ask concern these main courses. Studying these questions and their answers will enable us to understand the principles to follow when planning these central elements of our meals.

What are the best main courses for meals?

The word "best" of course may refer to many different things. To some people, it refers to quality; to others, taste; but, of course, in dieting, it should refer to the number of calories and to the fat content of a particular food item. For all people, whether dieting or not, the ideal main course is one that is basically protein and in which the protein is of high biological quality. For the dieter, we add an extra dimension in that this protein be also low in calories. Now, the easiest way to achieve this requirement in main courses is to select those proteins of high biological quality that contain the least amount of fat.

What is meant by "protein of high biological quality"?

The nutritive value of a protein really depends on the quality and quantity of the amino acids it contains. The amino acids are those parts of the protein that supply the ingredients for building new tissue. There are two kinds of amino acids, *essential* and *nonessential.* The essential ones are those that cannot be manufactured by the body and must be ingested. We need the nonessential amino acids also, but if not ingested, they can be manufactured from ingested amino acids by complicated chemical procedures within the body. The proteins of highest biological value are those that contain the largest number of essential amino acids. They are generally from animal sources and hence are called *animal proteins.*

Animal proteins are found in milk and cheese, eggs, meat, fish, fowl, and shellfish. In these foods the amino acids are supplied in about the same proportions in which they are needed by the human body.

Proteins of a lower biological value are those that are derived from fruits, vegetables, grains, and nuts. With a few exceptions they do not supply as good a variety of amino acids as those from animal sources. The outstanding exceptions among vegetable proteins are soy beans and chick-peas.

MEATS AND POULTRY

What are the best choices for the main-course protein for the dieter?

The best main course dishes for dieters are fish, shellfish, chicken, and veal. The less beef, lamb, and pork one eats, the quicker the weight loss. This is a very vital concept in dieting.

In my office, I always answer the question above by showing my patients a book called *Composition of Foods,** a publication of the U.S. Department of Agriculture known as *Handbook 8:* It is the most accurate source of calorie count and nutrient composition available, and is recognized as standard throughout the world.

In view of the high caloric content of beef, lamb, and pork, these are not the best choices for main courses.

A review of the meat items in *Handbook 8* reveals that with the

* Agriculture Handbook No. 8, available from the Superintendent of Documents, U.S. Government Printing Office, Washington, D.C. 20402, at $2.85.

exception of flank steak, which is the lowest-calorie form of beef generally eaten, the vast majority of beef cuts of choice grade have well over 1000 calories to the pound, with an average of about 1500 calories per pound. Prime grade beef (the highest quality) will have about 200 calories more than that. *Thus, most beef that is eaten contains approximately 100 calories to the ounce!* To visualize what an ounce looks like, visualize a meatball the size of a walnut. This is approximately one ounce of meat and, if of prime grade, it has about 100 calories. A pound of prime ribs of beef without the bone may run up to 2200 calories per pound! T-bone and porterhouse steaks run about 1600 calories to the pound, if of choice grade, and 1800 if prime.

Cuts of lamb of prime grade will run about 1200 calories to the pound. Lamb ribs run almost 2000 calories per pound. The lowest-calorie form of lamb is the leg of lamb, which averages about 1200 calories per pound when of prime grade. If you eat lamb, remember that every spoon of mint jelly that goes with it represents at least another 20 calories per spoonful.

Pork is the highest of all in calories. The tastiest pork, which is usually in the category of what is called the fat class, has almost 2000 calories per pound. Bacon alone averages almost 2700 calories per pound. After trimming, its average calorie count without bone or skin is about 1569 calories per pound. Except for spareribs and bacon, which are very high in calories, most trimmed lean cuts of pork average about 1500 to 1600 calories per pound, and those with less fat have about 1400 calories per pound.

Country-style, dried, or long-cured pork and ham are very high in calories; there are considerably fewer calories in the commercially light-cured and picnic cuts of ham. The lowest calorie count for pork products will be found in the canned and cured pork hams.

These figures will make it clear why beef, lamb, pork, and pork products are allowed for a maximum of only three dinners and three lunches per week on your diet.

When you do have beef or lamb, choose the leaner cuts such as flank and round beef cuts or the leg of lamb, and trim away all visible fat.

Why are beef, lamb, and pork cuts so high in calories?

The reason for this is their high fat content. Marbleization means fat! No matter how much fat is trimmed from the edges, the marbleization cannot be removed. Have you ever noticed leftover steak the day after it was originally cooked? Most people wrap their leftover steak in aluminum foil and refrigerate it. After it is cold, all of us have seen the little white spots on the meat and have noticed its greasy feel. These spots are, of course, fat which simply could not be seen when the steak was hot and the fat melted. This is equally true of lamb and pork.

Does it matter if both lunch and dinner include beef, lamb, or pork?

No, it does not matter as long as the total number of beef, lamb, or pork lunches do not exceed three per week, and the dinners also do not exceed three per week.

Incidentally, the restriction of three per week does not mean one may have three beef *and* three lamb *and* three pork, but three in total.

If one does eat steak, what is the best steak to eat?

The best, in terms of calories, means the lowest, and the steak lowest in calories is flank steak.

Are pickled meats allowed in the Diet Plans?

Yes.

Are corned meats permitted?

No.

Are smoked meats and smoked fowl allowed?

Yes.

May stews or potted meats with vegetables be eaten?

Yes, there would be no objection to this. The quantities of vegetables must be the same called for in your Diet Plan. In general, I suggest broiled meats since broiling allows the fat to drip off. (See pages 166–170 for food preparation questions.)

May cold meats be used for a nibble?

Meats vary from 50 to 125 calories, or even more, per ounce. A few ounces of meat brings a dieter's calorie count way out of line. In the Diet Plans, fruits are chosen for snacks because a whole fruit, which represents a lot of chewing, filling, and refreshment, rarely exceeds 75 calories per fruit. Never use meat for a snack!

How many calories add 1 pound to one's weight?

Approximately 3500.

Is tongue considered "beef"?

Yes, it is.

May wursts or sausages be eaten?

The problem with most of the wursts is that they have a very high calorie count since they consist of fatty pork products and often have extra fat added. Incidentally, many of them are quite salty and may result in the retention of some fluid, which is discouraging even though it does not add to the calories. Avoid all sausages except all-beef frankfurters and bologna, and keep those to a minimum. Remember, no salami and no liverwurst.

May luncheon meats be used?

No, they may not. Avoid these items inasmuch as their main ingredient is usually fatty pork. Also avoid corned beef and pastrami.

May meat products that contain a small portion of soybeans be used?

Yes, they may be used to the extent that any pure meat would be allowed on the diet.

What should be used in place of beef, pork, and lamb?

As previously indicated, the low-calorie foods in this category are veal, fish, shellfish, and poultry. As a group, these are considerably lower in calories than pork, lamb, and beef. In fact, it would take as much as five and six pounds of some fishes to equal the amount of calories in one pound of some of the beef and pork cuts. Interestingly enough, though a pound of beef always has more calories than a pound of fish, to make matters worse some people find they can easily eat more than a pound of beef, yet they consider a half-pound of fish as too much. More reason to avoid beef, lamb, and pork!

Why is veal allowed inasmuch as it really comes from a cow, as does beef?

Though it is true that veal comes from a calf or yearling, it is so young that the meat is not marbleized. All the fat that is present is on the outside of the meat, and can be easily trimmed off. It is assumed that the dieter will always cut all visible fat off *all* meats.

Which is better for the dieter, chicken or turkey?

Chicken does have fewer calories than turkey, though turkey has fewer calories than beef or lamb. A chicken fryer, ready to cook, has 325 calories to the pound. A roaster has about double this, as does a ready-to-cook turkey. The younger the turkey, the fewer the calories. Capons, hens and cocks, and fat, mature turkeys have about triple the calories of fryers—but do not fry the fryers!

Is there a difference between dark meat and light meat?

Yes, there is. There are fewer calories in light meat than dark meat. I do not consider the difference important.

May duck or goose be eaten in the Diet Plans?

No, they are considered on the forbidden item list. Even if the duck is made crisp, it is not allowed.

Should one eat the skin of a chicken?

No. The skin is too fatty, and should be removed, preferably before cooking.

Is game permitted for the dieter?

Most game is in the same caloric category as chicken, and there is no objection to including it (in the proper quantity that your Diet Plan calls for).

How does one handle unusual foods?

If one is on a foreign trip, or a friend serves something extremely unusual, it would be a shame not to try it just because it might be too fatty. These opportunities rarely recur, and should not be missed.

Are organ meats allowed on a diet?

Yes, but with one exception. Beef sweetbreads are forbidden, but otherwise all organ meats are allowed, and are considered rather low in calories. Some of them do have a high amount of cholesterol, so if cholesterol is your concern, do not eat a large amount of these meats.

Are chicken livers high in calories?

All liver is considered to be in the same category as the chicken–fish group, and is not regarded as falling into the beef group, regardless of the animal source of the liver.

What gravies should be used with meat?

None. Gravies are mostly thickened with flour. When natural, they usually contain a large amount of fat drippings, which is most easily noticed when the meat is cold and the fat congealed. Stay away from gravies when on a diet.

What condiments may be used with meats?

The condiments most often served with meats are ketchup, mustard, and steak sauces. The ingredients of some of these sauces are a secret formula so one can only guess at their allowability on a diet. Ketchup is not permitted on a diet, primarily because it contains a large amount of sugar, and, second, when people use ketchup, they tend to consume it by the tablespoon—often many tablespoons. I do allow mustard because mustard is used by the teaspoon and has very few calories. So far as the other steak and meat dressings are concerned, avoid those that appear to contain sugar. As a general rule, avoid those steak sauces you use by the tablespoon. If you are in doubt about a condiment, do not use it. I would have no objections to the use of those dressings that require only a small amount for taste, such as a few drops of Tabasco sauce.

FISH AND SHELLFISH

Must fish be eaten every week, and if so how often?

No. Fish is not required on the diet. What is required is that you do not have beef or lamb more than three lunches and three dinners per week. Therefore, one's choice must be either from fish, chicken, or veal. Learning to eat fish is one of the most important techniques in keeping weight down.

What are the lowest-calorie fishes?

The lowest-calorie fishes are shellfish, sole, flounder, and cod. There are about 358 calories to a pound of these fishes. At the other extreme, the highest-calorie fish is probably eel. Actually, we can divide the fishes into low-, medium-, and high-calorie groups. But remember, the highest-calorie fishes (unless they have been packed in oil) still have fewer calories than beef, pork, and lamb.

High-calorie fishes are as follows: anchovy (pickled), butterfish (northern), eel, herring (canned, plain, pickled, salted, smoked), lake trout (Siscowet), mackerel, sablefish, salmon (Atlantic, chinook), sardines (Pacific), shad (gizzard), Spanish mackerel, trout (rainbow).

The following are medium-calorie fishes: baracuda (Pacific), blue fish, buffalo fish, bonito, carp, chub, dogfish, halibut (Greenland), herring (Atlantic), jack-mackerel, kingfish, lake herring, lake trout, mullet, perch (white), pompano, porgy, salmon (chum, coho, pink, sockeye), sardines (Atlantic), shad (American), sheepshead, smelts, sturgeon, swordfish, terrapin, tuna, weakfish, yellowtail.

Low-calorie fishes and other seafoods are as follows: abalone, alewife, bass (all kinds), brook trout, bullhead. butterfish (gulf), catfish, clams, cod, crab, crappie, crayfish, croaker, flounder, frogs legs, grouper, haddock, hake, halibut (Atlantic and Pacific, California), herring (Pacific), longcod, lobster, muskellunge, mussels, ocean perch, octopus, oysters, perch (yellow), pickerel, pollock, pike, snapper, red horse, rockfish, sand dabs, sauger, seabass, shrimp, skate, snails, sole, squid, suckers, tautog, tilefish, tomcod, trout (brook), and turtle.

If the only fish on a menu is fried, which is preferable, beef or the fried fish?

The beef is preferable to the fried fish. If the choice were broiled fish *with a sauce,* choose the fish instead of the beef, and push the sauce aside.

May frozen fish be used on a diet?

Of course. In fact, frozen fish is very good for the dieter because it can be kept in the freezer at home and is always available as needed.

May canned fish be used?

Yes, if they are not canned in oil. Use fish canned in water, tomato or mustard sauces, but never eat fish packed in oil. The one exception to the rule is salmon packed in oil. It is allowed because it does not appear to absorb as much oil as do other oil-packed fish. Of course, it must be thoroughly drained. Incidentally, read labels carefully and avoid any sauces containing sugar. In situations where food choices are extremely limited, it is permissible, though not desirable, to use thoroughly drained and washed tuna that has been packed in oil. Oil-packed sardines and herring are impossible to drain adequately and should never be used.

Incidentally, there is marked variation among the different brands of water-packed tuna. If you do not like the taste of one brand, explore another one.

Is it allowable to have fish packed in soy oil?

No. From a caloric point of view *all* the oils are identical.

May I eat anchovies?

Anchovies are nearly always packed in oil. In this form they may not be eaten on the Diet Plans. Occasionally they are available packed in tomato paste, in which form they are allowed, if you can find them.

What about smoked fish?

Most smoked fishes are really dehydrated, or at least partially dehydrated, becoming so in the process of smoking. Inasmuch as the degree of dehydration varies from one fish to another and from the manner of processing, I have developed the general rule for all smoked fishes: If fish is smoked, use half the quantities called for in your Diet Plan. For example, if your particular diet calls for 4 ounces for lunch, you would have 2 ounces of smoked fish instead of the 4 ounces of regular fish as a full portion.

May gefilte fish (stuffed fish) be used?

There is no objection if it is *all* fish. However, gefilte fish is often made with matzo meal as well as sugar, and if so should not be used. If the contents are unknown, small amounts would be allowed for religious feasts, but always as part of the protein allowance of the main course. For example, if your diet called for 6 ounces of protein, there would be no objection to 2 ounces of fish and 4 ounces of meat.

What do you do if you hate fish?

This problem comes up more often than almost any other question. Try the many different types of fish available. Make sure that your market supplies *fresh* fish (if it tastes like cod liver oil it probably is not fresh). Modify the taste with lemon juice, wine, or tomato juice. Season with the many different herbs for new flavors. Try wrapping a piece of filet of sole around some shrimp and bake it with a little wine; even children like this. Try "diet sautéing," using onions, mushrooms, and broth instead of butter.

If you are willing to eat fish, you stand a good chance of getting used to it. If you get used to it, you stand a good chance of some day liking it. Believe it or not, when given half a chance, most people develop a taste for fish.

If I do not like fish, may I use shellfish?

Yes. Shellfish are very low in calories and an excellent main course for the dieter. Unfortunately, shellfish are high in cholesterol, so avoid their excessive use.

How do you measure portions of shellfish?

These are probably the most difficult foods of all to measure. Because shellfish are so low in calories, one need not be concerned if one's estimate is a little large. This does not mean that I advocate excessive portions. Avoid exceptionally large lobsters, but portion size in shellfish never is a real problem, with the possible exception of scallops (which are simple to measure) and shrimp.

How do you judge portion sizes of shrimp?

This is obviously difficult because of the large variety in shrimp sizes. Try weighing them at home on your postage scale to get an idea of their weights.

In general, these food items are so low in calories that if mistakes are made it rarely presents a major problem. But do not use this statement as an excuse to use larger portions than your Diet Plan recommends.

May the tiny canned Danish shrimp be eaten?

Yes, so long as they do not add up to more than the amount of protein allowed in your diet.

May caviar be used?

Yes, but remember that 3 teaspoons of caviar are equal to 1 ounce of meat. Make the appropriate arithmetical adjustment for this.

9

Vegetables and Salads

Many years ago I saw a cartoon in *The New Yorker* magazine in which a mother and little boy were walking down the street. The mother was describing what a good meal they were going to have for Thanksgiving. She said there would be an appetizer, a soup that her son particularly liked, turkey, stuffing, cranberry sauce, desserts, nuts, and so forth. The child's comment was, "Good, no vegetables."

One of the problems that many dieters have is that they never allow their eating habits to leave an adolescent level. One does not eat at age 6 as he did at age 1, or at age 16 as he did at age 6, so why should one at 46 be eating in the same manner as he did at 16? Perhaps now is the time for the dieter to up-grade his eating habits. You can open up new horizons, and the worst that can happen is that you will taste a food that you still do not like. Vegetables are a good food to start with. Let us go on to the questions most often asked about them.

Are vegetables important in a diet?

Vegetables are essential ingredients of a diet for a number of reasons. Primarily, they supply the body with required carbohydrates—the basic energy nutrient. Every vegetable does not supply an equal amount of carbohydrate; some supply much more than others. Vegetables are also an important source of essential vitamins, minerals, and bulk. Bulk in a diet not only gives one a feeling of fullness and satisfaction, but also allows for the intestinal action necessary for normal bowel movements. Constipation is a frequent problem in dieting, and an adequate bulk and roughage intake will help to prevent it.

Vegetables are a pleasant way to round out a meal and to add to its completeness. This feeling of completeness is highly beneficial psychologically.

What if I don't like vegetables?

Many of my patients say they don't like vegetables, and I have no reason to disbelieve them. I like to remind these patients of an experience that almost everyone can remember from our childhood: being invited to a friend's home for dinner and being served a vegetable that we did not like. Too embarrassed to tell our friend's mother, we would suffer through eating it, only to discover, much to our surprise, that we actually enjoyed the vegetable. We would then go home and ask our amazed mothers why they did not serve that particular vegetable. It has been my experience that if one *forces* himself to eat some new vegetables, more often than one would imagine he discovers that they are not so bad after all. You may, perhaps, also discover that you (or your wife) are really a better cook than your mother was.

If you do not like vegetables, explore anyway. Do not overcook them, and eat them while they are hot. Do not wait until you have finished all your meat and then complain that the vegetables are lukewarm and a little limp!

Does it matter which vegetables are eaten?

Yes, certainly. Vegetables should be divided into three categories:

1. Starchy vegetables. They are totally forbidden, and may *never* be eaten *while dieting*. The last two words are very important. This does not hold for eating after your proper weight is achieved. There is no lifetime prohibition on starches.

2. Cooked vegetables. Other than the starches, all cooked vegetables may be eaten, but only in defined amounts.

3. Raw nonstarchy vegetables. These may be eaten in unlimited quantity.

Which vegetables may be eaten, and how much of them?

All vegetables not on the forbidden list on page 103 may be eaten. Obviously not all at once, and equally obvious, only in controlled quantities. All cooked vegetables should be eaten in accordance with the quantities called for in the Diet Plans. Consider a half-cup as the standard measuring size for one portion. This is a volume, not a weight, measurement. Some vegetables, such as long asparagus stalks or broccoli, cannot be measured very easily with a measuring cup. In these cases estimate the quantity. Thus, a reasonable estimate for asparagus would be about six stalks.

Raw nonstarchy vegetables (except for raw green peas, which are forbidden) can be eaten in any quantity at any time. Use them as a green salad with meals, or as part of a sandwich, or as a base for a chef's salad meal, or as a snack between meals.

Why are the starchy vegetables forbidden and which are they?

The starchy vegetables are forbidden simply because they have too many calories. To allow them by the device of using extra-small portions is impractical and unrealistic. It is easier for the dieter not to have any. Do not eat any of the following:

Black-eyed peas	Macaroni*
Chick-peas	Noodles*
Corn	Pigeon peas
Cow peas	Potatoes
Dried peas	Rice
Kidney beans	Soybeans
Lentils	Spaghetti*
Lima beans	Yams

Are vegetarians healthier than nonvegetarians?

Not in my experience, but I am impressed with the care and attention that most vegetarians give to their food choices.

Why do some vegetarians have a weight problem?

Mostly because meals without animal protein, though filling during the meal because of bulk, have short durations of satisfaction. The nonvegetarian will often notice this after Chinese meals. There is then a tendency to satisfy the hunger by nibbling on hard cheese, which at 100 calories per ounce becomes the Achilles heel of the dieter.

* These, of course, are not vegetables, but inasmuch as so many people use them as such, I have included them in the list.

If one is a vegetarian can one have an adequate protein intake?

Yes, proteins are available to vegetarians, but it does require more care and more planning. Emphasis must be placed on an adequate amount of those vegetables which provide a high and varied quantity of protein, in order to insure an adequate supply of all necessary amino acids (the basic building blocks of proteins). If only one of the essential amino acids is missing, no matter what quantity of the other amino acids is available, the protein intake will be inadequate for the body's needs.

Some vegetarians avoid only some of the animal products and are perfectly willing to eat milk, fish, and eggs. Under these circumstances high-quality protein is readily available.

The vegetarian who eats fish is most fortunate, for in my opinion, ounce for ounce the highest quality protein probably comes from fish. Since less of each ounce is taken up by fat, more of it is devoted to protein.

The *total* vegetarian (often called a *vegan*), on the other hand, requires a high intake of the better vegetable sources of protein (soybeans, chick-peas, lentils).

May the same cooked vegetable be eaten every day?

No. It is a prime rule on these diet plans that a cooked vegetable should *never* be repeated two days in a row. Do not eat it on Thursday if you ate it on Wednesday, or know that it will be served on Friday. This rule gives the caloric balance required in these diet plans, provides a nutritionally sound vitamin and mineral balance and, equally important, the variety necessary to maintain interest in a diet program. Widen your food horizons and interests by pushing yourself into variety.

May vegetables be eaten with breakfast?

Yes, they may. Raw vegetables may be eaten freely. A cooked vegetable may be eaten in place of the slice of bread. A slice or two of tomato may be eaten as part of the allowance of one tomato a day.

May frozen or canned vegetables be used on a diet?

Certainly they may be used. The only real difference between canned and fresh vegetables is possibly in their taste and occasionally in their coloring. One word of warning: if the canned or frozen vegetables contain sugar, fats, oils, or butter, then they are not allowed. Read the labels carefully.

May dehydrated vegetables be used?

Dehydrated vegetables are a highly concentrated form of calories, in the dehydrated state. Therefore, do not use them in that state by sprinkling them on another food for flavoring. If these vegetables are used when fully reconstituted with water, they approximate the same caloric value as fresh vegetables. In general, dehydrated vegetables should be avoided unless fully reconstituted and measured after the reconstitution.

Are dried vegetables the same as "dehydrated"?

In the end result, yes, though they are processed differently. Because dried vegetables are usually served by the homemaker in quantities similar to those for regular vegetables, there is a tendency to end up with an excessively large caloric unit. The dieter should avoid dried vegetables on any weight-reduction program because of the difficulty they present in portion control.

How should vegetables be cooked?

Vegetables should be boiled, broiled, or baked. In fact they may be prepared in any way that does not require butter, cooking oil, lard, or margarine. Vegetables may be prepared in a nonstick pan without the addition of any fats. There is no objection to this kind of frying or sautéing. The most important thing is that absolutely under no circumstances should any fats *whatsoever* be added. Cheese sauces are equally incorrect and, of course, creamed vegetables are forbidden. Under no circumstances should sugar or honey be added (as in glazed carrots or beets).

Can vegetables be cooked without the use of butter and still be tasty?

First of all, successful dieting is usually based on accustoming oneself to a less fatty taste. The most important factor in vegetables, in terms of taste, is freshness and the avoidance of overcooking, which should always be guarded against. Use herbs and spices on vegetables for different flavors; for instance, try adding a few sesame seeds the next time you cook broccoli or spinach.

If quantities are carefully controlled, may any of the forbidden starches, such as a small baked potato, be eaten?

It is the rare individual who eats a *very small* baked potato. Have you ever seen anyone feel satisfied with a baked potato two inches in diameter? Obviously, it is possible to have such small quantities of these prohibited items that one can legitimately ask the question, "If I control the portion size why can't I include them?" Theoretically, you should be able to do so, but in reality this never happens. Starchy vegetables are invariably eaten in quantities too large for a diet portion, or too small for the dieter to feel psychologically satisfied. The caloric problem is further worsened by the fact that most people add butter or margarine to their potato or rice, or a sauce to spaghetti. And how many people will add sour cream to a baked potato! There is nothing sacred or magic about a baked potato. A potato is a potato! Baking it is better than frying it, but the potato is wrong to start with. And so are potato skins, no matter how well scraped. Stay away from potatoes in any form.

If you have a digestive problem, of course, and starches have been specifically prescribed, potatoes may be used, but be extremely precise in portion control. Use a half-cup as a standard measuring unit for a portion, and never add butter or other fats. It will throw the calorie count off somewhat, and may result in a slightly slower weight loss.

Is there any way to add potato to the dinner meal?

No. However, this does not hold true with young children on a diet, and in special circumstances when there may be gastrointestinal disease or food allergies.

Since the Chinese in China tend to be so thin, and they live on rice, what is wrong with rice on a diet?

First of all, the Chinese use rice as the major food staple and do not eat the other fattening foods that we eat. Rice is only a small part of our diet. The problem with rice is similar to the potato problem. Rice is high in calories, people tend to eat it in large quantities, and almost invariably they will add a fat to it. A typical advertisement will always show a bed of rice with a pat of butter melting over it. The only circumstance in which rice is permitted is when you are using it as a substitute for a cereal. Otherwise, no rice!

Is there any caloric difference between white and brown rice?

No.

May rice be used instead of cereal?

Yes, if measured carefully (use a half-cup as a full portion). Remember, use skimmed milk only with it.

May green peas be eaten at all on the diet?

Yes, but only as a cooked vegetable in the half-cup portions called for on your Diet Plan. Do not eat raw peas; as a high-calorie finger food they are too dangerous!

Why are green peas allowed?

Green peas are a higher-calorie vegetable but not as high as those on the forbidden list. They are allowed in a controlled portion of a half-cup. Dried peas of any type are not allowed.

Are beets allowed on a diet?

I am questioned about beets more than about any other vegetable. Beets are a very good vegetable, and are allowed on a diet. Many people become confused and concerned because they think of beet sugar when they think of beets. Beet sugar comes from a specific type of beet not used as a cooked vegetable. There is absolutely no objection to eating boiled beets as one of your vegetables. Actually, they are fairly low in calories. The only form of cooked beets that are not allowed, of course, are glazed beets, in which honey and sugar are used. Incidentally, cold boiled beets are a good vegetable for those summer months when cold meals seem more appropriate. Avoid pickled beets as they often contain added sugar.

May sauerkraut be eaten on a diet?

Yes, sauerkraut is allowed even though some people do make it with a small amount of sugar. Actually, I never knew sugar was used in its preparation until I recently saw commercially canned sauerkraut in which artificial sweetening was used. Consider sauerkraut a raw vegetable. If you are sensitive to a high-salt intake, however, remember that this is a high-salt vegetable.

May I have corn on the diet?

No. Corn is a high-calorie food, served in large portions, and usually eaten with butter if on the cob, or with cream sauces if not on the cob.

May I have white radishes on a diet?

Yes. Any kind of radish is allowed by the same rules, as long as they are either raw, or in the cooked form, in the half-cup amounts allowed on your Diet Plan.

Are baked beans allowed?

No!

Can pickled tomatoes be used?

Yes, but subject to the general limit of no more than one tomato a day.

May I truly have endless amounts of carrots?

Yes, so long as they are raw. Obviously, this could be carried to a ridiculous extreme. Moderation and reasonableness must enter into your judgment.

Prolonged overeating of carrots, or of any yellow fruits and vegetables, such as pumpkin, may result in a condition known as carotonemia. This is a condition in which the skin gradually turns an orange-yellow in color. It is first seen in the palms of the hands. It is not dangerous, but not particularly attractive.

May I eat Jerusalem artichokes?

Yes, as a vegetable, but I do not suggest the use of bread made from Jerusalem artichokes.

Are vegetables counted when used in a stew?

First of all, do not include any vegetables on the forbidden list (potatoes, etc.). If a quarter cup or less per person is used, it is safe to ignore the quantity. If a quarter to a half cup per person is used, consider the stew to contain one vegetable serving. If three-quarters to a full cup per person is used, consider the stew to contain two vegetable servings.

What do I do about vegetables in restaurants?

Look for those vegetables that are less likely to require butter, and always ask if they can be prepared for you without butter. If this is not feasible, follow these rules: If there is an obvious excess of butter, simply do not eat any cooked vegetables at that meal. If there is a minimum of butter, eat the vegetable in spite of the fact that it was cooked with butter.

Must one have a salad with every meal?

No, but it is a nice addition to have.

Is tomato a vegetable or a fruit?

Technically, it is a fruit, but most people eat it as a vegetable. There are some special rules that I use for tomatoes:

> Tomato juice may be used freely in cooking. It is limited to a 4-ounce serving as an appetizer; it may be used in 6-ounce units as a fruit substitute.
>
> One is limited to one whole medium-sized tomato in salads, or sliced in a lunch sandwich.

One may use a half cup of cooked tomato as a cooked vegetable portion.

One may use a whole tomato as a substitute for another fruit.

May I add raw vegetables to breakfast?

Yes, there is no reason why you cannot add raw vegetables to this meal.

Need salad be measured?

No. It may be eaten in any quantity.

Why do the Diet Plans allow all the raw vegetables you want, but limit the amount of cooked vegetables? Aren't the calories the same?

A pound of raw vegetables has exactly the same calories before cooking as it does after cooking. The major reason for allowing unlimited raw vegetables and limiting the amount of cooked vegetables is the fact that when vegetables are raw there is really a limit to how much chewing one will do, whereas when vegetables are cooked and soft, less chewing is required and many people consume excess quantities without conscious awareness. Just visualize how few raw string beans or carrots fit in a half cup but how many cooked string beans and carrots will fit in a half cup when they are soft. Incidentally, excessive raw vegetable intake may cause an uncomfortable degree of flatulence (intestinal gas), which in turn forces one voluntarily to control the amount of raw vegetables eaten.

Are all raw vegetables allowed?

Absolutely any raw vegetables other than peas. Of course the obvious ones are lettuce, cucumber, and radishes, but there is nothing wrong with having raw string beans, asparagus, mushrooms (I don't mean canned mushrooms—anything that has been canned has been cooked), green peppers, carrots, celery. If it is a vegetable, you can eat it raw. Try raw zucchini, broccoli, and rutabagas also. Raw spinach and mushrooms make a wonderful salad.

How many calories are there in commonly eaten raw vegetables?

The vegetables most often eaten raw contain the following calories:

Vegetable	*Approximate number of calories*
1 carrot	42
3 carrot sticks (each 3 in. long and ⅜-in. thick)	13
2 olives	13
4 leaves of lettuce	13
1 tomato (small)	22
1 stalk of celery (large)	9

May I use the unflavored gelatins in salads?

Yes. Tomato juice also may be added, if desired, to make an aspic.

Instead of having one vegetable at dinner may I use oil on my salad?

No! Absolutely not. Use your diet, not only to lose weight, but also as a learning period to become accustomed to nonoily, nonfatty tastes. This is a very important concept in dieting. When you are finished with your diet, you should be able to use oil in your salad dressing, but you will be using smaller amounts. The more accustomed you are to nonfatty tastes, the better off you will be.

What are the best low-calorie dressings to use?

The best dressing for the dieter is vinegar and/or lemon juice. The use of salad oil is specifically forbidden. Nonabsorbable oil, such as mineral oil, may be used in very small quantities, but its use has the disadvantage of furthering the desire for oily tastes and, if used in too large quantities, it may cause diarrhea. It may also interfere with the proper absorption of oil-soluble vitamins.

There are some commercial dietetic dressings available, but read the labels very carefully. Unless the dressing contains *3 or less calories per teaspoon,* do not use it. If you use a proper low-calorie dressing, avoid its excessive use. A convenient and tasty dressing can be prepared by purchasing a commercial type that comes in small packages, and in which you are supposed to add the vinegar and oil. Follow the instructions except where they state that you should add oil, and instead replace the oil with tomato juice.

Here is a recipe for diet salad dressing that many patients have enjoyed:

Diet Salad Dressing

½ cup tomato juice
2 scallions
1 tablespoon lemon juice
1 teaspoon parsley
¼ teaspoon salt
Dash of Tabasco
Dash of pepper

Finely chop the scallions and the parsley. Combine all the ingredients in a jar with a tight-fitting lid. Cover and shake well to blend ingredients. Store in refrigerator. Shake well before using. Makes about ½ cup.

May I have wine vinegar?

Yes.

May soy sauce be used on a diet?

Yes, it certainly may. If you are a water retainer,* be careful of the quantity you use, inasmuch as soy sauce has a very high salt content.

If I am dining out, and the salad is already made with oil, should I eat it?

I would strongly recommend that you do not eat it. I think it is more important that you do not have the oil than to have the salad.

May a fruit be used in place of a vegetable?

Occasionally, it may be appropriate to serve a fruit such as apple or cranberry sauce (made without sugar) or a mixture of rhubarb and

* An increased salt intake often results in an increased retention of water. When the body excretes the additional salt, it also excretes the additional water. Some individuals appear to be more sensitive to minor changes than others. Most women are particularly susceptible to retaining salt, and consequently more water, just before their menstrual periods. This water retention is recognized not only by a sudden weight increase, but often also by a feeling of bloating, slight swelling of the ankles, occasional puffiness around the eyes, and a tightness of one's finger rings.

cranberries in place of a vegetable. There is no objection to this occasional substitution. However, avoid fruits in green salads. They add extra unnecessary calories. Save fruits for dessert. And at festive meals where small crab apples or spiced peaches are served with the main course, they should be avoided inasmuch as they are usually prepared with sugar.

10

Fruits

Among the most important items in the Diet Plan are fruits. They mainly supply carbohydrates and, as I have said before, carbohydrates are an essential part of a healthful diet. Carbohydrates are the major source of immediate energy. Recent studies on athletic stars have shown that maximum energy for athletic performance can be achieved by overworking the individual a day or two before the big contest, and by filling him with a high amount of carbohydrates immediately before the event. This gives the muscles a maximum supply of chemical energy. For this purpose fruit is better than steak.

In order that you do not go through a diet without adequate energy, include the full amount of carbohydrates listed in your Diet Plan. Carbohydrates are limited in quantity on the diet as a caloric control.

Other important reasons for eating fruits are that they are important sources of vitamins and minerals, and supply bulk that the body must have. Fruits—in amount indicated on your Diet Plan—are excellent snack foods. They are also a very good form of dessert. Dinner desserts are particularly useful on a diet and should not be skipped. The dessert provides a definite psychological benefit for many people in that it marks the end of a meal. Those diners who do not have a dessert often end up picking, picking, picking, whereas once a dessert is eaten it winds up the meal conclusively, particularly if eaten along with a cup of tea or coffee.

The questions asked by my patients show that there are many facts about fruits that dieters often misunderstand. Let us consider these questions and see what the facts are.

Are citrus fruits really important?

Citrus fruits (oranges, grapefruits, tangerines, etc.) are important because they are the single best source of vitamin C. You should definitely have one citrus fruit a day, unless you are allergic to them. Make it a habit to have it at breakfast every day, and then it is unnecessary to remind yourself about it later on.

Which has more vitamin C, the fruit or the juice?

There is no difference.

Instead of citrus fruit for breakfast, may I have another kind of fruit, including berries?

Yes, but on the condition that one of the fruits during the remainder of the day is a citrus fruit.

Won't grapefruit help me lose weight?

I do not know who started the grapefruit myths, but there is no extra value to grapefruit. It is simply another citrus fruit with more vitamin C than other such fruits, having somewhat fewer calories in proper portions than most other fruits, but without any magical capability of burning calories. If you enjoy grapefruit, eat half of one as a fruit portion, but do not expect it to work magic.

What does one do if he is allergic to citrus fruit?

Avoid this group and have your physician prescribe vitamin C, which should be taken daily.

What fruits are really the lowest in calories?

The lowest are: gooseberries, apricots, grapefruit, loganberries, peaches, pumpkins, and strawberries.

May lunch or dinner be started with a fruit?

No. Of course, the calories are the same if you take a fruit at the beginning or at the end of a meal. Psychologically, however, there is more satisfaction in having the fruit at the end of a meal. Use tomato juice as a starter if you wish. If there is a very special circumstance you may start dinner with a fruit, but you must skip the dessert at that meal!

May fruit be eaten with cottage cheese for lunch?

Yes, but use the fruit as a substitute for one slice of bread. The fruit may be melon (other than watermelon), other fresh fruit, or *water-packed* canned fruit.

May berries be used?

Yes, berries are allowed. They are a delicious, low-calorie fruit. Use them with the skimmed milk from your allowance, if you desire.

What fruits should not be eaten on a diet?
Are there any fruits that are really bad for you?

The first rule is to stay away from those fruits whose quantity you cannot control. Examples of these are watermelon, grapes, and cherries. Very few people could eat only a dozen grapes or cherries. I call these finger foods, and once one starts eating them he often goes on and on until the bag or dish is empty. In fact, in most families, whoever discovers the bag of grapes or cherries in the refrigerator is often the *only* one to eat grapes or cherries; before one realizes it, the whole bag is gone. Incidentally, this points up another rule in eating. This is the rule of never eating unless you are sitting down. If you have fruit on a plate, seated at a table, you will eat much less than if you stand at the open refrigerator and pick one cherry after another. Stay away from cherries, grapes, and raisins.

Why shouldn't watermelon be used on a diet?

Only because if you like watermelon, the average portion eaten tends to contain between 300 to 500 calories! There are few watermelon lovers who will settle for a piece of watermelon three-fourths of an inch thick, a quarter round! Most watermelon eaters will eat wedges, or half rounds, two inches thick. It is not unusual for a watermelon portion to contain over 300 calories.

What if watermelon, grapes, or cherries are part of a fruit cup? Should they be picked out?

No. I have no objection if these items are in a fruit cup. The reason I forbid these items is because of the difficulty in controlling quantity. If the total content of the fruit cup is restricted to a half-cup, there is no objection to the individual ingredients.

Are there any other "forbidden fruits"?

Yes, there are. As with vegetables, do not eat any dried fruits. This includes prunes, raisins, figs, dates, apples, apricots, peaches, pears, pineapple, or dried fruits of any type. They are too high in calories per "satisfying unit volume." Glazed fruits are also forbidden. Also, avoid olives and avocados, both of which have a high fat content.

Though it is easy to see why fruits packaged in sugar are not allowed, what is wrong with dried fruits?

Dried fruits are dehydrated, and without their normal water content they are a very concentrated source of calories. Prunes are, after all, dried plums, and the plums used to make the prunes are usually large-sized fruit. Now ordinarily in the diet we might allow one medium-sized plum, or two small plums, or possibly three very small plums, such as the little Italian plums, but it is very easy to eat three, four, or even five prunes. This is the same as eating five very large plums. Consequently, on a diet one should stay away from all dried fruits. This includes the juice of these fruits too. Fig and grape juices contain too many calories for the dieter. Also avoid prune juice unless you need it to relieve constipation (see also page 202).

What should I know about very rare and unusual fruits?

Obviously no list can be so complete as to include all fruits. Use your judgment if you eat the following ones (or other fruits not included here).

Acerola	Low in calories
Amaranth	Low in calories
Breadfruit	High in calories
Granadilla	High in calories
Guava	Medium in calories
Haws	High in calories
Kiwis	Medium in calories
Loquats	Medium in calories
Plantain	Very high in calories
Pokenberry	Low in calories
Sapodillo	Very high in calories
Sapotes	Very high in calories
Tamarind	Very high in calories
Ugli fruit	Medium in calories

What is the correct size of a fruit portion?

The basic size of a fruit is a whole, medium-sized fruit. Stay away from the very large fruits, what I call the "bon voyage size." Of course, there is no need to settle for miniature ones either. Judging the size of fruits requires honesty. If you are in the market and are not sure whether a particular fruit is too large or medium, consider it too large and take a smaller one.

Fruits may be mixed: For example, one may have half an apple and half a pear, or a quarter each of a peach and pear, and half an apple. However, when you start eating raw fruit in wedge form, there is a problem. For example, if one was given a large bowl of fruit wedges, one would be likely to eat more than the equivalent of one whole fruit. This is a psychological thing. When you eat very tiny pieces of food, there is a tendency to eat and eat, whereas a whole fruit defines itself in size.

Some fruits such as grapefruit, or even big papayas, are obviously very large. For these, use half a fruit as a full portion. Some fruits, such as pineapple, must be used in slices or wedges. Estimate the size equivalent to a half cup. If the fruits are in very small pieces, as in a fruit cup, consider a half cup as a portion.

The specific portions for each fruit are as follows:

Fruit	*Portion*
Apple	1 medium (2½-inch diameter is the maximum size allowed; be careful since many apples are larger than this size)

Apricot	3 small *or* 2 medium
Banana	½ medium (this will be a better choice than a whole banana, no matter how small)
Berries	½ cup
Blackberries	
Blueberries	
Boysenberries	
Cranberries	
Currents	
Gooseberries	
Loganberries	
Mulberries	
Raspberries	
Strawberries	
Dates (fresh)	2
Figs (fresh)	2 medium
Grapefruit (pink or white)	½
Kumquats	5 medium
Lemons	2
Limes	2
Lychees (raw only—if you can get them)	3
Mango	½
Melon:	½ small
Cantaloupe	½ small
All others (except watermelon):	
Cranshaw	2-inch wedge
Honeydew	2-inch wedge
Persian	2-inch wedge
Spanish	2-inch wedge
Nectarine	1 medium *or* 2 small
Orange	1 medium (2¾ inch diameter is the maximum allowed)
Papaya	½
Peach	1
Pear	½ medium *or* 1 small
Persimmon	½
Pineapple	1½ slices
Plums	2 small
Pomegranate	1 medium
Pumpkin	½ cup
Quince	1 medium
Tangerine	1 large
Tomato	1 medium

Are there any general rules for fruit size?

A correct portion is the following:

2 fruits, if very small (e.g., apricot)
1 fruit, if standard (e.g., apple, peach)
½ fruit, if very large (e.g., grapefruit, papaya, pear)
½ cup of very small fruits (e.g., berries, fruit salad)
½ small cantaloupe; 2-inch wedge of other melons (except watermelon)
1½ slices of pineapple

Is there any problem in having half of a large cantaloupe if a small cantaloupe is not available?

If you have a large cantaloupe, eat a quarter instead of a half.

Are there less calories in a peeled apple than in an unpeeled apple?

Only to the extent of the little amount of apple one leaves with the peel. This is not enough to make any difference.

May canned fruits be used?

No, because they contain added sugar! Water-packed fruits, however, are allowed.

Why can't canned fruits be used if they have been washed?

They should not be used because the sugar in which almost all canned fruits are cooked actually gets into the fruit and develops an equilibrium with it. The fruit itself has more calories than it had before it was canned because of the additional sugar. Washing cannot take off all this sugar. If only canned fruits are available, use only those that have been canned *without sugar*. Read those labels carefully. In many *dietetically* canned fruits the sugar has simply been reduced rather than eliminated. Use only those that have no added sugar. If you are in an absolute trap and there is no way out of using fruit canned in sugar or syrup, then make sure it is washed in very hot water, very thoroughly. Sugar does dissolve more easily in hot water than in cold water. Then chill it in the refrigerator after washing. This is not ideal, but it is a way of dealing with a difficult situation. The water-packed varieties of canned fruits, with or without artificial sweetening, are tougher to find than regular ones, but your grocer can get them for you.

May I use fruit packed in its own juice?

Yes, but the juice must be thoroughly drained off. After all, the juice represents extra calories.

Are frozen fruits permitted?

Frozen fruits are of two types. One of them is packed in sugar. They are absolutely not permitted. The other frozen fruits are not packed in sugar. These are allowed in the same way that any raw fruit is. Read your labels!

May cooked fruit be used on a diet?

Any approved fresh fruit may be cooked as long as sugar is never added. Artificial sweetening may be used in cooking if desired, but cooked fruit often tastes better if it is added after cooking. One of the great tricks that was discovered by the Department of Health of the City of New York, was the use of noncaloric soda beverages as a sweetener for baked apples. Try black cherry or raspberry, pouring it over the fruit instead of using sugar. Incidentally, there is one other great tasting baked fruit that people rarely ever mention, baked pears. These are made in exactly the same way you would bake an apple. Pineapples and grapefruits can also be prepared in this manner.

One word of warning: Many people use very large apples for baking. If you do, consider half an apple as a fruit portion. And never order a baked apple in a restaurant. They are always prepared with sugar.

Apple sauce, cranberry sauce, and rhubarb are interesting fruit variations, but must be prepared without sugar. Use artificial sweeteners for necessary sweetening. When used in half-cup portions, they are all low-calorie food items.

May fruit juice be substituted for fruit?

Yes, it may. Most dieters find it more satisfying to chew things. But if you wish to have fruit juice, there would be no objection. Consider all fruit juices in 4-ounce units as equal to a whole fruit. And of course if it is canned, if it is packaged, *watch those labels!* Never, never use juice sweetened with sugar. Even unsweetened grape juice and prune juice or the nectars (apricot, peach, pear) are not allowed.

In place of a fruit in the afternoon, may I have a glass of tomato juice?

You may have an unsweetened juice in place of your fruit. Be sure to use 4-ounce glasses for all but tomato juice, which is allowed in 6-ounce quantities when it replaces a fruit.

11

Milk and Milk Products

Milk may well be the most important single food item in anyone's diet. It is the near-perfect food, for it is high in most of the required nutrients. Milk is a wonderful source of protein, minerals, and vitamins. It is also certainly the best single source of calcium, and calcium is required, not only during the growing years, but throughout life. One quart of milk supplies more calcium than three dozen eggs. Milk is also the richest source of riboflavin, and a quart of milk provides more protein than five ounces of beef. In fact, milk contains all the elements of the perfect food except for iron, vitamin C (this is lost in pasteurization), and vitamin D, which today is usually added to milk, including skimmed milk.

Although no single food is absolutely essential, since a substitute can be found for everything, milk should form part of everyone's diet except in unusual circumstances (see page 127). It is not only highly nutritious, but it is also an excellent filler and an appetite appeaser. Drink milk—it is a positive asset for success in your dieting.

Another unusual advantage of milk is that in the countless different forms of cheese it offers wide variety and tempts the palates of many who prefer to eat it in that form.

Now let's take up the facts dieters want to know about milk and milk products, as shown by their questions.

MILK

What are the best kinds of milk to drink?

The only milk to be used on a diet is skimmed milk—milk that is 99.9 percent fat free—or fat-free buttermilk. Buttermilk is really the milk left over when the butter is taken out. (Hence the name buttermilk; those little pieces floating in buttermilk are not butter.) Today it is made by adding lactic acid bacteria to skimmed milk, and is therefore called cultured buttermilk. In theory, there is no difference in the number of calories found in buttermilk and in skimmed milk, but in actual practice, most milk processors add butterfat to the buttermilk, and therefore I do not allow buttermilk on my diets unless it is known to be fat free. If you cannot obtain fat-free buttermilk, you can make your own with skimmed milk and some commercial buttermilk as a starter.

Skimmed milk has all the characteristics of whole milk except for its lack of fat and its lower amounts of vitamins A and D. Most milks today are fortified by having vitamins A and D added. In these milks the calcium and other minerals, as well as the protein, milk sugar, and water-soluble vitamins are exactly the same as in whole milk. It makes no difference whether one uses powdered skimmed milk (you reconstitute it by adding water) or the liquid skimmed milk. Some processors add some extra skimmed-milk solids to skimmed milk to give it a richer taste. This will add somewhat to the calories, but not enough to make a significant difference.

If you wish to use the powdered skimmed milk, which is very inexpensive, there are some tricks that you should know. Powdered skimmed milk takes a little while to mix well with the added water. Mix it very thoroughly and leave it in the refrigerator overnight before using it. People who do not like skimmed milk made from powder tend not to like it because it is either not mixed well or not cold enough. Another less expensive way of buying milk is to purchase evaporated skimmed milk, which is prepared for use by adding an equal amount of cold water.

What are the correct amounts of milk for dieters?

Most adults and teen-aged girls should drink two 8-ounce glasses of skimmed milk daily. If this is not feasible, the dieter should consider one 8-ounce glass as an absolute minimum. Teen-aged boys should drink three glasses a day and consider two glasses as a minimum. Preteen dieters, both boys and girls, should drink three glasses daily.

When is the best time to drink milk?

The timing is really a matter of personal choice and somewhat dependent upon one's life style, as well as on when one is hungry. For some, milk fits in best at meal times, particularly lunch or breakfast. For others, milk is a great snack food when taken in the afternoon or at night before going to bed. There is no nutritional or weight-loss advantage to having one's milk at any special time of the day.

I really cannot stand skimmed milk. It looks blue instead of white. Must I drink it? Can't I substitute a smaller amount of whole milk or at least use the 99 percent milks?

The main reason for the use of milk in the skimmed form is that it is the lowest-calorie milk there is. But there is another reason almost as important. Switching to skimmed milk is part of the learning process of adjusting to nonfatty tastes. After a while almost everybody gets accustomed to skimmed milk to the point where if they drink whole milk in error, they will say, "It tastes like cream." Often getting accustomed to the taste takes only a few weeks.

Without fat, the milk really is thinner. It is this thinness that gives skimmed milk its bluish color.

There are preparations of fluid skimmed milk and skimmed milk powder containing dietetic chocolate flavoring. These contain almost no additional calories, and I have no objection to using this chocolate-flavored milk. One must be careful, however, that the label does not read "chocolate drink." This means it is a combination of milk, chocolate flavoring, and water, with not enough milk to label it as such. Chocolate drink does not have enough food value for dieting purposes.

What is wrong with the 99 percent milks or the 2 percent milks?

Answering this question really requires a definition of terms, and in particular the comparative percentages of fat in the various forms of milk. Whole milk (the "regular" homogenized milk that is most popular) has an average of 3.6 percent fat, or, in other words, is 96.4 percent fat free. The following chart shows the fat characteristics of the different milks:

Type	*Percent fat free*	*Percent fat*	*Approximate calories per 8-oz. glass*
Whole milk	96.4	3.6	170
2 percent milk	98.0	2.0	132
99 percent fat free	99.0	1.0	110
Skimmed milk	99.9	0.1	85

This chart makes completely clear the reason why skimmed milk, with its much lower fat content, is preferable on a diet.

May I have my full 16 ounces of milk at one sitting?

Consider the eating day as having six eating units: breakfast, mid-morning snack, lunch, mid-afternoon snack, dinner, and evening snack. Do not exceed 8 ounces in any one eating unit. You may have less ounces per unit, but never more than 8 ounces at any given time.

Must milk be used in 8-ounce portions? Is there any objection to using 2-ounce portions of milk six to eight times, or 4-ounce portions three to four times?

No, there is no objection at all. One must simply be careful that the measurements are correct.

What is a "skim-shake"?

The "skim-shake" is a tasty, filling drink, particularly if milk is not one of your favorite foods. Simply mix your milk with some low-calorie soda, or add a few drops of vanilla extract or a little instant coffee, and put it in a blender. This is particularly nice as a bedtime drink.

May I use my skimmed milk allowance in cooking?

There is no objection to this.

Who should avoid milk?

1. Those who are allergic to milk. Some persons who are allergic to fluid milk, however, are occasionally able to take other milk products, but usually in small quantities.

2. Anyone who tends to have diarrhea from milk. This may be related to quantity. Recently we have learned that many people lack an intestinal enzyme, lactase, that helps to digest the natural sugar in milk; this may be the reason for chronic digestive disturbances in large numbers of persons.

3. Those who have such a severe aversion to milk that it is truly offensive to them. There is no need to be a martyr.

May sour cream be used on a diet?

Believe it or not, there is not the least difference in the amount of calories between sweet cream and sour cream. We have heavy sour cream, medium sour cream, and light sour cream, the same as we have heavy sweet cream, medium sweet cream, and light sweet cream. These are all, whether they be sweet or sour, *very* high-calorie substances and there is no room for them in a sensible diet program. Stay away from them. And remember, people who use sour cream on their potatoes will rarely use just a tiny bit. One ounce (two *level* tablespoons) contains 57 calories!

CHEESE

Are all cheeses the same to the dieter?

No. Cheese can be classified into three groups, soft, hard, and cottage cheese.

Soft cheeses. These are the cheeses that one spreads with a knife, such as cream cheese. They are high in fat, lower in protein, and are difficult to measure because they are usually used as spreads. Therefore I do not allow them. Avoid the "dietetic" soft cheeses also.

Hard cheeses. These are the cheeses that one cuts with a knife, whence the name *hard cheese.* They are easily measured, and are often purchased precut into slices. Read the package label or weigh the cheese on your postage scale to make sure of the weights.

Cottage cheeses. These are the high-volume cheeses, and are generally low in calories and form an important part of a dieter's food allowance.

What are the best hard cheeses to use?

There is no such category as the *best* hard cheese. A few hard cheeses are made from partially skimmed milk, but it is very difficult to determine the exact amounts, and I do not feel that there is a significant caloric difference in most instances.

Hard cheese is a convenient food for a sandwich. You may also eat it plain, possibly with a little mustard. Or, if you wish, have a melted cheese sandwich (using no butter, of course).

May cheese be used as a main course for dinner?

Yes, it may. Control the quantity carefully. If you choose cottage cheese, you are allowed double the number of ounces you would be allowed if you chose meat or fish for the main course. If you choose a hard cheese, use half the number of ounces you would be allowed if you had meat or fish for dinner.

May I add Parmesan or other cheeses to my meats?

Yes, if you measure carefully, and eliminate 1 ounce of meat for each half-ounce of cheese used. For example, if one is entitled to 6 ounces of meat as a dinner portion, the portion may be changed to 4 ounces of meat plus 1 ounce of cheese. It is essential that the portions be carefully controlled.

Are meat-cheese combinations allowed?

Technically, yes. The "technically" really refers to your ability to measure the ingredients. Avoid these combinations away from home. Cheeseburgers are a good example of how one can get into trouble with combinations.

A cheeseburger is really a hamburger *plus* a slice or two of cheese. No commercial cook ever takes away part of the hamburger when he adds the cheese. That slice of cheese can represent an unnecessary, additional 75 calories. Teach yourself to have a hamburger *or* a cheese sandwich at lunch, not a cheeseburger.

How do you measure food combinations, such as meat and cheese?

If you make sure to measure carefully, you may replace *each ounce* of meat, fish, or poultry on your Diet Plan with one of the following:

½ ounce of hard cheese, *or*
1 ounce of farmer cheese, *or*
2 ounces of cottage cheese, *or*
1 egg (but do not exceed 2 eggs at a meal, or 4 eggs per week)

There is also no objection to any mixture of meat, fish, or poultry so long as the total ounces do not exceed your Diet Plan allowance for that meal.

May cheese be used as a dessert?

Yes, it may. Simply substitute three-fourths of an ounce of hard cheese for your fruit. If you are honestly careful in your portion control, you may use half a cheese portion together with half a fruit portion.

Is cheese safe to use for a "nibble"?

No. Most hard cheeses have 100 calories per ounce. Though a highly nutritious food, such cheese is also a high-calorie food. A few pieces of cheese eaten as a nibble can add up to over 300 calories. Therefore, no!

Must skimmed milk cottage cheese be used?
Is creamed cottage cheese allowed?

Today, there are many varieties of plain cottage cheese, all of which are allowed. Theoretically, all cottage cheese is made from skimmed milk, but to improve the taste, most dairies cream it, which includes the addition of some whole-milk product. The undesirable taste of uncreamed or skimmed-milk cottage cheese mostly results from the fact that it is usually salt free. The addition of a little salt will often give it a very nice flavor. In general, I suggest one use the partially creamed, or so-called diet-type cottage cheeses, but I do not object to the use of creamed cottage cheese if that is all that is available.

Are pot, farmer, or ricotta cheeses allowed?

Yes, they are. They are variants of cottage cheese. They are used in the same portions as cottage cheese, except for farmer cheese. Most farmer cheeses today have a higher fat content, and therefore should be used in portions half the weight of the cottage cheese portions allowed on your Diet Plan.

Is cottage cheese with premixed fruits and vegetables allowed?

The answer to this would depend on the exact brand you are using, and what its actual calorie content is. If the calorie count exceeds 30 calories per ounce, do not use it.

YOGURT

Is yogurt a helpful food on a diet?

No, I don't think it is. In fact, I find that many manufacturers of yogurt advertise it in such a way that to some extent people are really misled. For example, almost all the advertising for yogurt as a diet food is done with a lot of emphasis on how few calories plain yogurt contains. When yogurt is discussed from the point of view of taste, just as much emphasis is put on the fact that it comes in a variety of fruit flavors: strawberry, prune, pineapple, and so on. Thus, one goes into a store thinking of how few calories plain yogurt contains, but at the same time recalling how tasty the fruit yogurts are—and one usually buys the more fattening fruit-flavored yogurt. Actually, many of the fruit-flavored yogurts have 100 calories more per container than does the plain yogurt, or the equivalent of over 5 to 6 teaspoons of sugar!

The story on yogurt is as follows: Much of the yogurt sold today is made from half whole milk and half skimmed milk, and therefore has a calorie count halfway between whole milk and skimmed milk. (It is very difficult to obtain yogurt made purely from skimmed milk unless you make your own at home.) Some yogurts are made from whole milk. All yogurt is simply a different culture of milk. I like to call it milk that you eat with a spoon which has a somewhat soured taste. It has all the same food values as milk, and of course contains the same number of calories. Because of the sour taste, however, many people prefer to have it sweetened. It can be sweetened with plain flavors such as coffee or vanilla which add about forty calories more to the 8-ounce container of yogurt. When it is sweetened with fruit, however, it will often have some 100 to 120 calories more than the plain yogurt. Most manufacturers cite their calorie count as being 135 calories for an eight-ounce container of plain yogurt, about 180 calories for the simple flavors, and 260 calories for the fruit-flavored ones. Though I have not seen it recently, in the past some manufacturers have sold a fruit-flavored yogurt that was made with artificial sweeteners; this, of course, kept the calorie count down considerably. If you can find a fruit-flavored yogurt that is made with artificial flavoring instead of sugar, then I would have no objection to 4 ounces of it being used as a dessert. If you love yogurt and are willing to eat the plain variety, use a 6-ounce portion of plain yogurt as equivalent to a 4-ounce serving of ice cream.

May I eat yogurt as my entire lunch?

No. Yogurt is only a form of milk and cannot be used as a meal.

12

Eggs

Eggs are a good source of protein, which we want; a high source of fat, which we do not want; a low-calorie, satisfying food, which we want; and a high source of cholesterol, which we do not want. Eggs are a good food, but must be used judiciously.

How many eggs is it safe to have?

I suggest that people restrict their egg intake to about 4 eggs a week. This is not for calorie reasons; it is not for weight reasons; but, rather, is one of the devices to help lower the blood cholesterol level. This is not an absolute requirement, but a prudent measure for good health.

May cottage cheese, or hard cheese, be mixed with eggs for a cheese omelet? May it be used as a dinner meal?

Yes, if you are in control of the portions used. If your lunch called for a meat or fish portion of 3 ounces, you could have 2 eggs together with half an ounce of hard cheese or with 2 ounces of cottage cheese. Dinner would call for larger portions if desired, but, for cholesterol reasons, do not exceed two eggs at a meal.

If I don't like whole eggs, may I have the whites or the yolks separately?

The whites of eggs are allowed. As a matter of fact, you are allowed two whites for every regular egg on the diet. The yellows (yolks) are not allowed separately at all.

May I use the low cholesterol egg substitutes?

By use of these new products, you may have more than 4 eggs a week. You may substitute one egg portion for each egg on the Diet Plan, even though these egg substitutes have about 25 calories more than a natural egg.

May something other than eggs, cheese, or cereal be eaten for breakfast?

Yes, you may have fish or poultry in 2-ounce portions.

13

Breads and Cereals

I am sometimes asked why breads are included in a diet, since they can be fattening if consumed to excess. Bread is probably the most maligned item of food there is, for if eaten in moderation it is a food with a high degree of nutritional value, particularly the whole-grain types. Bread is very satisfying and it is an extremely convenient food since it allows people to eat sandwiches, which in our culture often makes the difference between being able to stick to a diet or not. It also does not have so many calories that it cannot be well controlled. Bread is a good food. *It belongs on a diet!*

The questions often asked by my patients about bread reveal some common misconceptions and problems that I shall try to clear up.

BREADS

What are the best breads to use?

The best breads are the whole-grain or enriched breads, thinly sliced.

Must breads be thinly sliced?

When available, this is the most desirable type of slicing.

How much difference does it make if bread is thinly sliced?

This is a matter of arithmetic. Most breads are cut into slices that weigh 1 ounce each. The average bread slice has about 70 calories. The black breads such as pumpernickel, however, very often have molasses added to give them the black color (and the sweeter taste). These breads have more calories per ounce and therefore are not permitted on a diet. Bread is an important element of a diet, having both a nutritional and a practical function. For most dieters, the ideal slice of bread averages about two-thirds of an ounce. Whether they are called protein bread or by any other name, the so-called low-calorie breads have less in calories simply because they are cut thinner. Most thinly sliced breads will average anywhere from 39 (the extra thin) to 50 calories per slice. Use thinly sliced bread whenever it is available. In other words, stick to these breads when you are home or if you bring a sandwich to work or to school. Do not use the full-thickness breads *unless* you are away from home and the thinner slices are unavailable. If you have doubts about the bread you use, if the label says "thin sliced" but a slice feels heavy, weigh it on your postage scale. A thin slice should not weigh more than two-thirds of an ounce.

Is it worthwhile substituting a half slice of bread if thinly sliced bread is not available?

I do not think this is necessary. One rarely gets the same psychological satisfaction from using a half slice of bread as one does from a whole slice of bread, no matter how thinly sliced. That is why I recommend using the thinly sliced bread at home.

If you are having cereal for breakfast, do you also have bread?

No, when you have a cereal no bread should be eaten for breakfast, unless you are on a Diet Plan which calls for it specifically.

Does it matter if bread is toasted?

No, it does not matter.

Is there any objection to rye bread?

No, but in some parts of the country rye breads are sliced very thickly and contain less air. There is no objection to rye breads if one is certain that each slice weighs no more than 1 ounce.

Are sandwiches advisable on a diet?

If your Diet Plan allows one slice of bread, it means an open sandwich, while the two slices of bread on many Diet Plans permit a closed sandwich. I find it actually preferable to eat sandwiches for a diet lunch. It is the easiest way I know to control, at lunch, the quantity of the main course, which is where the majority of lunch calories are found. After all, how much meat can respectably be put on a slice of bread? A hamburger that looks adequate in size on a hamburger roll rarely looks adequate on a plate alone. One will be satisfied with smaller meat portions if the sandwich form is used.

May melba toast, rye crisps, zweiback, or matzo be used?

These items do not have the same nutritional value as most enriched or whole-grain breads, and in the long run I think the standard bread slices serve the dieter's purposes better. I see no objection to using these items occasionally. Note there are brand differences as well as possible changes by the manufacturer in the size of the portions! I suggest the following equivalency usage, but check the box labels first.

One slice of bread of full thickness equals:

4 long melba toasts
⅔ matzo square
3 rye crisps
1½ zweiback

One thin slice of bread equals:

3 long melba toasts
½ matzo square
2 rye crisps
1 zweiback

What breads should be avoided?

Avoid the pumpernickels, cornbreads, muffins and, ordinarily, bagels. From a nutritional point of view, whole-grain breads, of course, offer you the most food value. So far as bagels are concerned, for those people who are on a very rigid cholesterol-control diet and must avoid all kinds of shortening, a bagel is a good bread because it has no shortening.

May I substitute a half a bagel for a slice of bread?

Formerly, almost all bagels were about 2 ounces in weight and their average caloric content was about 135 calories. Today, bagels often weigh 3 ounces or more. I have seen bagels weighing as much as 4 ounces. A 4-ounce bagel, of course, would contain about 300 calories, and half of a 4-ounce bagel 150 calories. Since a thin slice of bread has less than 50 calories, the difference in calories between this and half a bagel can be large. This is why I do not suggest eating half a bagel. If the bagel is *so* important to you, arithmetically one could have a quarter, or a third of a bagel, but obviously this is not at all satisfying psychologically. Also, bagels are not enriched. There is considerably less food value in them than in the regular slices of enriched bread.

May muffins be used?

The problem with muffins is, of course, the same as with bagels. They are large, and the caloric value of half a muffin would depend, of course, on the muffin's actual weight. The ideal technique for the dieter is to stick to the plain breads, thinly sliced.

May popovers or biscuits be used?

No. These are both very high in calories. In fact, some nutrition books classify a popover as a pancake. Do not be fooled by the big air spaces. These breads are loaded with calories.

What about rolls?

In general, the water rolls have fewer calories than soft rolls, and considerably less than sweet rolls. Rolls are usually made of highly milled flour and are rarely enriched. Consequently, their nutritional value is low, though their calories are high. Often they weigh much more than 1 ounce. Therefore, I do not allow any rolls except hamburger and frankfurter rolls.

Why are hamburger or frankfurter rolls allowed?

Only for convenience. Count half a roll as equal to a slice of bread and use rolls only with frankfurters or hamburgers. There is no need for you to ask for regular bread when you are eating a hamburger.

If I have a frankfurter, isn't it really better to throw away the roll?

You need the carbohydrate of the roll as much as you need the protein of the frankfurter, and believe it or not, there are more calories in the frankfurter than in the roll.

If I miss breakfast, may I have a roll and butter at the office?

Do not miss breakfast! If the diet is important enough, get up in time. If you cannot get the correct food, do not eat the wrong food. If you are totally trapped, as when you are a guest for breakfast, and the food served is not on your diet, eat a half portion.

What about other breads: French, Italian, Syrian, Norwegian, flat breads, tortillas, etc.?

Obviously there is no way to make a list to include *all* specialty breads. Most of these breads may be used if their weight is known. Use two-thirds of an ounce as an equivalent to a thin slice, and 1 ounce as equal to a full slice. The most important consideration is the purpose for which the bread is used. The main advantage of bread is its use for sandwiches. Very few of these specialty breads are suitable for sandwich making.

Must I pick the raisins out of raisin bread?

No. The calorie count of raisin bread is about the same as that of other breads.

May bread sticks be substituted for bread?

Bread sticks are difficult to control in terms of weight. After all, how many bread sticks are there to the ounce? And remember that bread sticks vary from the thin, long Italian type to the stubby ones with sesame seeds. They are also a nibble food, and dieters *must* learn to avoid nibble foods totally. Therefore, do not use bread sticks!

How about bread sticks made with Jerusalem artichokes?

These really serve no valid purpose. There is insufficient calorie saving, and as bread sticks they promote nibbling.

If in traveling there is no way to get a protein for breakfast, may two slices of bread or a roll be substituted for the protein?

No. In those circumstances I would simply do without the protein. It is better to do without a little than to break the diet pattern. In the long run, weight maintenance is mostly determined by the eating patterns learned during dieting.

May crackers be substituted for bread?

No. There is inadequate nutritional value and inadequate satisfaction in the small amount that would be allowed. One Ritz cracker has almost as many calories as a lump of sugar, and did you ever notice how greasy your fingers feel after picking up the cracker? Even one of those small triangle things, or wheat thins, has 9 calories, and a Triscuit has even more calories than a Ritz cracker.

May dry soda crackers be used to control morning sickness in pregnancy?

Under these circumstances, I would suggest two dry, unsalted soda crackers soon after arising. Have your breakfast somewhat later and omit the bread at this meal.

CEREALS

Cereals are basically grains, and therefore are considered with breads. Cereals are eaten either hot or cold. Most of the hot cereals are high in nutritional value and may be used at breakfast in half-cup (cooked) quantities. Either the regular, five-minute or instant types may be used.

Cold or dry cereals are of varying nutritional value. Some have been so depleted of vitamins that about the only value you get from eating the cereals results from the milk that accompanies them. Other cold cereals are of higher nutritional value and make a pleasant alternative food for breakfast. Use cereal either by the individual packet serving, or by weighing out up to 1 ounce. Do not go by volume. Some cereals, such as Grape-Nuts, Familia, Granola, etc., are rather dense cereals and there is a tendency to use much too much of them. Stay away from these when dieting.

What may one use with cereals instead of milk?

First of all, let me say that any milk used with cereals must be skimmed and must be counted as part of your daily allowance. If you do not like milk, try cereal with orange juice. Yes, orange juice! Sounds peculiar, but some people do like it that way, though it might take a few separate servings to get accustomed to it. And, of course, there is no reason why dry cereal cannot be eaten dry!

14

Desserts

If your Diet Plan calls for desserts, eat them. Strictly speaking, they are optional, but you will be better off if you eat them. They add a basic sense of completion to a meal, which is very important psychologically.

Are the alternative desserts in the Diet Plans as satisfactory as fruit?

Yes. The three basic alternative desserts are three-quarters of an ounce of hard cheese, *or* a portion of dietetic gelatin, *or* a portion of ice cream *or* ice milk. I have been allowing my patients ice cream and ice milk for over 20 years without any interference with their dietary success. I include them because they are nice dessert foods, a good milk substitute, and a welcome little treat to have, particularly at a time when one is feeling somewhat deprived by the diet. Ice cream is sold by fluid volume; that is, by the half-pint, pint, quart, or gallon. Actually, its cost depends for the most part on its bulk weight. The reason why one make of ice cream is expensive and another inexpensive can be figured out easily at the ice cream freezer of the supermarket. Take two equal containers of ice cream, one of the high-priced variety and one of the low-priced brand, and hold one in each hand. You will be amazed at what a marked difference in weight there is between the inexpensive and the expensive one. The higher the quality of the ice cream, the heavier it is. It is heavier also because there is more ice cream and less air per unit volume; therefore it will contain more fat. Higher-quality ice creams always contain more fat and less air. Most states have laws regulating how much fat must be present in order for the substance to be legally labeled ice cream.

From the caloric point of view, therefore, the cheaper the ice cream the better off you are. The correct portion on a diet is a serving of 4 ounces by volume (note that with ice cream we make an exception and use volume rather than weight measurement). In other words, the correct portion is a quarter-pint. If you include ice cream on your diet, give up both one glass of skimmed milk and one fruit for that day. Do this no more often than three or four times a week. But don't feel guilty if you are eating ice cream. It is a healthful food and so long as you are using it as a substitute for milk and fruit it is a fair exchange. Better yet, use ice milk instead of ice cream. Ice milk has a less fatty taste, sometimes a somewhat sweeter taste. It is a nice thing to have on a diet and contains fewer calories than ice cream. Use it in the same amounts.

Is ice milk preferable to ice cream? How do they differ?

Ice milk is similar to ice cream, but it has a lower fat content. Some of the ice milks have a little more sugar than does ice cream, but there are more calories in fat than in sugar, so ice milk usually contains fewer calories than ice cream. Interestingly, a high-quality ice milk may have more calories than a very cheap ice cream, because of the high air content in the cheaper ice cream. On the whole, although I do allow ice cream for the dieter, I recommend ice milk.

What are the best flavors of ice cream?

As mentioned previously, *best* can refer either to taste or to calories. Here we are talking about the calorie problem. I suggest that you stick to the plain flavors, such as vanilla, coffee, or chocolate. Yes, I said chocolate! Avoid those flavors that have nuts in them because of the higher calorie content given by the nuts. Also avoid flavors containing pieces of chocolate, such as chocolate chip, and the various fudge ice creams.

Is dietetic ice cream better?

No. The term *dietetic ice cream* usually refers to ice cream made without sugar for diabetic patients. Its fat content is as high as that of regular ice cream, but it has somewhat lowered caloric value because it is artificially sweetened. Unless you are a diabetic, you will be better off eating ice milk than the dietetic ice cream. There are more calories in dietetic ice cream than in ice milk, and not much less than in regular ice cream of similar fat content.

How many calories are there in a cone for ice cream?

There are 45 calories in the cone itself!

How many calories are there in the chocolate covering of a chocolate-covered ice cream bar?

There are about 30 calories!

May the ice cream allowed on the diet be added to coffee?

I suggest that it not be, since I really think people should get used to black coffee. If you truly do get an upset stomach from black coffee, then I suggest you use in your coffee the skimmed milk from your milk allowance. Besides, most dieters will get more satisfaction from eating a dish of ice cream than from drinking part of it in their coffee.

May ice cream be substituted for alcohol?

No. Ice cream is in a food category, alcohol is in the alcohol category. Alcohol is allowed as an extra, over and above one's daily food requirement. There is an adequate allowance of ice cream on the Diet Plans for most people's taste and social needs. The additional allowance of alcohol entitles one to alcoholic beverages exclusively. The caloric value of the alcohol is not transferable to other foods. If you do not drink your allotment you are simply staying fully on the Diet Plan. After all, though allowed, the alcohol does add calories to the Diet Plan.

May soft ice creams be substituted for ice cream?

Yes, but be sure their labels actually use the term *ice cream*. Otherwise they may not have sufficient food value to replace one milk and one fruit serving. There is usually a large amount of air in the soft ice creams, and they are on the low side in fats.

What do you do if you can't control the amount of ice cream or ice milk?

Some dieters are almost hypnotized by ice cream and ice milk and go through the constant self-torture of having just another spoonful. I can't count the number of my patients who will go through a pint, or quart, even a half-gallon of ice milk, saying, "Just another small spoonful." If this is a problem for you, then do the following: *Do not bring ice cream or ice milk into your home.* Instead, save your ice milk- or ice cream-eating experiences for when you are in restaurants where you would be too embarrassed to order a second dessert. But remember, if you have an ice cream cone, throw away the cone itself, since it has 45 calories. *If* you are afraid of temptation, purchase a Dixie cup. And certainly avoid the chocolate-covered ice cream pops with their high-calorie casings.

Is sherbet preferable to ice cream?

No. I prefer that sherbet not be used. Basically ice cream and ice milk are used in the Diet Plans as milk substitutes. Most sherbets, even though some contain enough milk to be labeled milk sherbet, do not have enough milk to make a suitable milk substitute for the purposes of the diet. Though sherbets contain fewer calories than ice cream, they have considerably less nutritional value, and therefore are not appropriate for a diet.

Is there any objection to water ices?

Yes, there is. In general, almost all of the ices available consist strictly of sugar, water, and flavoring; they are high in calories and low in nutritional value, and are out-of-bounds for all dieters!

May the low-calorie diet gelatin desserts (such as the D-Zerta brand) be used on the diet?

Yes, as a fruit substitute. Do not use the diet gelatins as an extra food, even though they are so low in calories. This is because one should get accustomed to not having more than one dessert at a meal.

May the low-calorie diet puddings (such as D-Zerta brand puddings) be allowed on the diet?

Yes, the puddings made with skimmed milk from your milk allowance may be used in place of a fruit.

If I really feel that I just must have some cake, is there any serious objection to a very tiny piece of plain pound cake?

Everybody thinks that pound cake, because it is "plain," is the lowest-calorie cake. Actually, it is one of the higher-calorie cakes. According to the U.S. Department of Agriculture, it contains over 2000 calories to a pound! Yes, over 2000 calories! That tiny 2-ounce sliver has 250 calories! Do not take even a crumb of this cake on your diet. By using the terms *sliver* or *tiny* you are simply fooling yourself.

How many calories are there in other cakes?

While the cake highest in calories is probably the previously discussed pound cake with its 2000 calories to the pound, the lowest is probably angel food cake with about 1200 calories per pound. Frozen devil's fool cake might run about 1700 calories per pound, and a simple sponge cake about 1300 calories to the pound. Cupcakes have about 1600 calories to the pound. The average commercial cupcake weighs from 1 to 2½ ounces, which means they have from 100 to 250 calories per cupcake! The average slice of pound cake weighs from 1½ to 2½ ounces, and thus has from 175 to 300 calories per slice! No matter what the circumstances, no matter what the urge, do not eat that piece of cake! No matter how thin the sliver is, it has too many calories.

Are cheese cakes made from cottage cheese allowed?

No, they are not. The total caloric count is too high, and secondly, the eating of any cake defeats our purposes of creating new diet patterns. To develop a new style of eating requires teaching oneself to avoid cakes and pastries.

Is there anything wrong with nibbling on nuts?

Yes, there is! Remember, these are very fatty foods. Most of the nuts are basic suppliers of oil. Do not eat any kind of nuts or seeds while on a diet. The only time I do not mind the use of seeds is when they are used in small quantities and sprinkled on food for flavor, as with poppy seeds, caraway seeds, or sesame seeds. In general, though, nuts and seeds are *finger foods,* and as mentioned before the major problem with finger foods is that there is no stopping. It is impossible not to have a second peanut after having the first, and so on. The only way not to eat peanuts is not to have the first peanut. This holds equally true for all other nuts.

What about dietetic candy?

Dietetic candy should not be eaten for two reasons. First, it does have some calories, and, second, you are simply encouraging yourself to keep on putting something into your mouth. One of the important techniques in weight loss and weight control is teaching yourself to keep things out of your mouth.

Can licorice be eaten on a diet?

No!

How can I resist an especially tempting dessert?

This is a good question, as well as a crucial one, with which to end the section on desserts. It does present a true dieting dilemma. The answer to it must be partly psychological and partly philosophical. The choice is really between immediate gratification and your long-term goals. To be thinner, you really need a kind of special purpose. If you succumb to this need for immediate gratification, then obviously the goals get pushed further and further away. On the other hand, when you begin to recognize *and accept* that the long-term weight-reduction goals are real, are important, and are of long-lasting benefit, then and only then will the need for immediate gratification become less important.

It helps in resisting such temptations to imagine yourself, as you are, fully undressed in front of a mirror, and then visualize exactly how you would *like* to look. Remember, whether you will be thin or fat is *your* choice.

There must be a very firm realization that what you eat today determines what the scale will show tomorrow. Too many people forget the simple, direct relationship between today's weighing and yesterday's eating.

An important attribute of maturity is the ability to postpone immediate gratification. It is upon this type of maturity that much of anyone's success in dieting depends. You resist the dessert if it is important enough to you to be thinner, *if the taste of thinness tastes better than the taste of the dessert!*

15

Snacks: What To Do If You Are Hungry

An important concept to remember in dieting is that if you are hungry during a meal (or immediately before a meal), the probability is that no matter how intense the hunger feelings are, these feelings will have disappeared within 20 minutes after you have eaten. If you will wait out those 20 minutes, your hunger will be forgotten. Snacks are primarily provided for those between-meal periods when your hunger may persist.

Some persons almost want the world to stop turning when they are hungry. Almost nothing will interfere with their desire to get something to eat, and the quest for a snack becomes a terribly important one. At the same time, all of us have been in situations such as being stuck on the road in a traffic jam or with a flat tire at a time when we were very hungry with absolutely no access to food. Somehow we all manage to put up with these situations and survive them, ultimately without unreasonable discomfort. Though I do not ask my readers to be Spartans, I do expect them to understand that at times it is difficult not to be somewhat hungry.

The between-meal snacks in your Diet Plan are calculated as part of your weight-control program. Not eating them will not accomplish any great saving, whereas eating them, particularly in the late afternoon, may result in the avoidance of fatigue and irritability which may be the consequence of a relative hypoglycemia (lowering of the blood sugar). This hypoglycemia is not a disease state but a normal occurrence in anyone who has not eaten for a while.

As mentioned earlier, snacks are primarily allowed whenever the meals are more than four hours apart, and, therefore, for most people, they are allowed between lunch and dinner and before bedtime.

May a fruit snack ever be eaten in the mid-morning?

Not ordinarily, but there is one exception. If there is a six-hour or longer time span between breakfast and lunch, then one should have a snack during the morning. If one does this, then one must give up the mid-afternoon or the late-evening snack.

What snacks are allowed?

There are two types of snacks that are allowed: a limited group and an unlimited group.

Limited Group

Most Diet Plans call for a snack in the mid-afternoon and in the evening. This primarily refers to a fruit portion. If you wish, the following substitutions are allowed in place of one fruit:

2 oz. cottage cheese
¾ oz. hard cheese (no crackers)
2 oz. fish
1 egg or the whites of 2 hard-boiled eggs
Dietetic gelatin

Unlimited Group

This group refers to raw vegetables, which except for raw peas may be eaten in any quantity and at any time. There is no limit to the amount of raw vegetables that may be consumed.

What is the "maximum vs. optimum" theory?

For some dieters, the phrase "without limit" appears to trigger some unrealistic thinking. Many people look at a diet almost as they would a legal contract. In return for their agreement to stay on the diet, they wish to eat absolutely everything that they are enitled to. In other words, they feel that if it is coming to them they should eat it. Sooner or later, one must accept a more mature attitude about this and recognize that the best way to diet is to eat the optimal amount that will provide for weight loss and appetite satisfaction, not the maximal amount. This is true, not only of snacks, but also of the sizes of portions of the other foods included on the diet.

Is cold chicken satisfactory as a snack?

If you feel you can get the same satisfaction from 2 ounces of chicken as from a fruit, I would have no objection.

Will I lose weight faster if I do not eat any snacks?

Technically, the fewer calories one eats, the quicker one should lose weight, but good dieting is a balance between losing weight and feeling comfortable. There is no need to eliminate snacks totally but, on the other hand, it would serve no purpose to force yourself to eat a snack if you have no desire for one.

May I skip a snack in the afternoon and have two in the evening?

No, you should not do this. If you skip a snack, consider it permanently gone. Never have a second snack in the evening except in special circumstances.

What are the special circumstances in which I may have a second snack in the evening?

This is primarily for people in college and living in dormitories. Dormitory life is usually associated with extra evening eating as well as going to bed at very late hours. A second snack will often make the difference between success and failure on a diet for the college student.

The only other time an extra snack is allowed is if you stay up to an excessively late hour beyond midnight.

May beverages be used as snacks?

One may drink any noncaloric beverage at any time and in any circumstance, without limit. You may also drink your skimmed milk at any time, but never exceed the quantity you are allowed for the day.

May I chew gum if I am hungry?

I strongly recommend that people do not chew gum while dieting. Gum chewing is another oral technique very closely allied to chewing food. Basically, the overweight individual should learn to use his mouth less often—in other words, put fewer things into his mouth. Every time such a person chews gum he is simply repeating one of the basic actions that has gotten him into trouble: chewing, chewing, chewing. If, however, you feel you must chew gum (sometimes people who have recently given up cigarettes find this is their only sure way of staying away from cigarettes)—if you *absolutely must* chew gum, and I emphasize the words *absolutely must,* then, of course, stick to one of the sugar-free gums. They do have some calories, but less than do the regular gums.

If I take up smoking, will I eat less?

Just because people respond to giving up smoking by eating more does not mean you will eat less if you start to smoke. Under no circumstances should you start to smoke to avoid snacking. It will not help.

How does one control snacking after smoking marijuana?

Some of my patients describe smoking marijuana as being followed by a sensation known as the "hungries" or "munchies." Marijuana is said to result in a sensation-expanding experience which may include the sensation of hunger. In reality, after speaking to many of hundreds of patients who have used marijuana, the so-called increase in appetite is mostly a matter of mind over matter. It is absolutely possible to control your appetite after having smoked marijuana. If you *must* snack, choose the correct snack foods (see page 148). If you are unable to control your eating, don't smoke!*

---

* While I feel I should answer this question realistically, that doesn't mean I advise the use of marijuana, possession of which under present laws may land one in prison for years.

16

Spices and Condiments

Spices and condiments with which to add extra zest and flavor to your food are allowed in the Diet Plans, but with some exceptions. Use soy and Worcestershire sauces, mustard, vinegar, or curry powder. Do *not* use ketchup, chili or tartar sauce. Cocktail sauces for shellfish should be avoided because they have a ketchup base, but Tabasco and horseradish may be used.

Spices that are sprinkled on may be used freely. They will add a taste variety to your diet, so do explore the large number of spices available.

A general rule for spices and condiments is: When used normally as a pinch (as with dill, onion powder, parsley, etc.), or by the drop (vanilla extract), or by the teaspoon (mustard), they are allowed, but when they are used by the tablespoon (ketchup, tartar sauce, etc.), they are not permitted.

Is salt forbidden when dieting?

Unless your doctor has put you on a low-salt diet because of a particular medical problem, I know of no reason, just for the sake of weight reduction, that one should be on a salt-free diet. Use salt freely, but remember that an excessive use of salt may result in some water retention which, in turn, can be quite discouraging when reflected on the scale. If you are a water retainer then moderate your salt intake.

Contrary to an impression some people have, it is not necessary to restrict one's salt intake to get started on a diet. The decrease in your total food consumption will automatically result in an adequate, natural reduction in salt.

Are salt substitutes allowed?

Yes, but do not use them unless your doctor prescribes them.

May these diets be followed if you are on a salt-restricted diet?

Yes, they may, but certain modifications should be made. The degree of modifications will depend upon the degree of salt restriction. *Discuss this with your doctor.* Certainly avoid table salt, salty spices (garlic salt, celery salt, onion salt, etc.), pickles, sauerkraut, and broth and bouillon.

May imitation butter flavor be used?

Absolutely not! One of the goals of this diet is to have the dieter get some new sets of tastes—nonfat, nonbuttery tastes.

May chili be used?

Chili powder may be used, but chili as a bean dish may not be eaten.

What flavorings are allowed?

Almost any flavoring that is basically used in units of a few drops or no more than a teaspoonful. Vanilla extract is a good example of this. Avoid those flavorings that give very intense sweet tastes, such as artificial maple syrup.

Are pickles allowed?

Pickles are allowed in any reasonable quantity at any time, except for the sweet or gherkin pickles.

17

Vitamins and Minerals

The Diet Plans in this book are all adequate in vitamins and minerals if you use variety in your choices of foods. If you run the risk of inadequate variety, I suggest that you take a daily vitamin supplement composed approximately as follows:

Vitamin A—10,000 units	Vitamin B_6—2.5 milligrams
Vitamin D—400 units	Vitamin C—100 milligrams
Vitamin B— 5 milligrams	Niacinamide—25 milligrams
Vitamin B_2—5 milligrams	Vitamin B_{12}—2 milligrams

Are therapeutic vitamins better than multiple vitamins?

Therapeutic vitamins are of higher dosage than the multiple-vitamin formula suggested above. It is not necessary to supplement the Diet Plans with high-dosage vitamins; they are an unnecessary expense and offer no medical advantage. Therapeutic vitamins should be used on a physician's specific order to treat a specific vitamin lack or nutrition disorder.

With what meal should vitamins be taken?

It doesn't matter. Most people take their vitamins with breakfast simply because it is easier to remember, and they are always home for breakfast.

Should the vitamins have added minerals?

Added minerals are generally unnecessary, but I would have no objection to your using them.

Do vitamins increase your appetite?

No, I do not think that vitamins increase the appetite in a well-nourished individual.

Is it necessary to take potassium if you are on a diuretic, while dieting?

This is something you should ask your physician. High-potassium foods (e.g., oranges) are included in your Diet Plan, but do not exceed the quantities your Diet Plan allows.

18

Nonalcoholic Beverages

Liquids are an essential part of one's dietary intake. Thirst represents a drive which is even stronger than hunger. No diet discussion can be complete without answering the many questions that pertain to one's fluid intake.

What nonalcoholic beverages are allowed?

Water
Plain soda water—club soda, not sweet soda
Lemonade or limeade, if artificially sweetened
Dietetic sodas (those without any sugar)
Tea
Coffee, including decaffeinated coffee
Skimmed milk in the amounts called for on your Diet Plan.

When are these beverages allowed?

They are allowed at any time with one exception: Avoid using any sweet beverage to accompany your main dinner meal. In general, I find that the dieter develops better eating habits if he does not drink sweet soda drinks *with* dinner, even though it is sweetened artificially and not with sugar. It tends to make all foods taste sweet. Use water or milk with your meals, not dietetic soda.

Are there any beverages that should be avoided?

Avoid any beverage that contains sugar. This even includes dietetic soda that has some sugar. The rule for dietetic beverages or, in fact, for any beverage, is to allow freely only those beverages that have *no more than 1 calorie per ounce.*

Also avoid coffee substitutes such as Postum and cocoa because they contain too many calories.

How much water should I drink?

The amount of water you drink is purely at your own discretion, depending on thirst. There is no magic or special advantage to having an exact number of glasses of water daily, as some diet writers have advised. Remember, the body in its own wisdom maintains a constant balance between the lavatory and the faucet. What comes in must go out. Let your thirst be the guide.

Is there any limit on the amount of dietetic soda that one may drink?

In view of the indecision on the part of the U.S. Food and Drug Administration as to the safety of artificial sweeteners, I feel that to insure safety, one should limit oneself to a maximum of two 16-ounce bottles of dietetic beverages per day.

If one is at a party and only regular soda drinks are available, can this be an exception?

Absolutely not. If there is no dietetic beverage available, one usually can find plain soda water (club soda). Try adding some lemon or lime. And, of course, it is rare for plain water not to be available.

Are commercially prepared, frozen or fresh limeade and lemonade allowed?

Only if they contain no sugar.

How much tea or coffee may one drink while on a diet?

I do not feel that there is any limit on the amount of coffee or tea that one may drink. Obviously when I say no limit, I am not expecting anyone to go beyond the limits of prudence. To take so much tea or coffee that one is jittery, cannot sleep at night, or has a digestive disturbance is not acceptable. Some individuals avoid these problems by using decaffeinated coffees. It does not matter if the coffee is brewed, instant, or freeze-dried. The coffee and tea may be hot or iced. If you use the prepared brands of iced tea, read your labels carefully and choose only those brands without any sugar. They are available.

All tea and coffee must be black—unless there are specific medical reasons to the contrary, never use any lightener, regardless of type!

The reason behind all this is to save calories, many calories, during maintenance, and also to adjust yourself to nonfatty tastes. If you drank three cups of coffee daily and added 1 ounce (2 tablespoons) of light cream (also known as coffee or table cream), you would be consuming 180 calories a day, the equivalent of about 18 pounds of body weight in a year. The chart below shows the yearly calories consumed by an individual using 1 ounce of various lighteners in 3 cups of coffee daily, and the body weight that could be lost if they were not consumed:

Lightener	*Calories in 1 oz.*	*Calories in 3 cups daily*	*Weight (in lbs.) represented by these calories in 1 year*
Light (coffee or table) cream	60	180	18
Half-and-half	40	120	12
Whole milk	20	60	6
99% fat-free milk	15	45	5
Skimmed milk	10	30	3

Obviously, if you like your coffee dark, you will consume fewer calories. On the other hand, if you prefer your coffee light, or have more cups of coffee, such as second cups after various meals, or extra coffee at coffee breaks, you will consume considerably more calories if you add a lightener.

When one looks at the chart, it is very easy to say that there are very few calories in an ounce of skimmed milk, but remember, those 3 pounds a year that you can save also mean *you can save 30 pounds in 10 years!* Even if you take only skimmed milk in your coffee, what happens when you visit a friend or eat in a restaurant, and skimmed milk is not available? The individual who is accustomed to having skimmed milk in his coffee will almost always use cream rather than have it black when skimmed milk is not served.

The way to avoid these problems is simply to force yourself at first to drink your coffee black. Do not replace it with tea. Even if you cannot swallow more than one sip, that is all right. But do it again and again. Before long you will manage to swallow two sips, then three sips, and before you know it you will be a black-coffee drinker. The average length of time this takes most of my patients is 3 weeks—not very long for a lifetime habit change.

Teach yourself to drink your coffee black. It is worth the effort, as thousands of patients will testify. It is a habit that once learned, stays with you forever. The biggest problem about becoming a black-coffee drinker is that you will be much more demanding about the quality of your coffee.

Why shouldn't artificial or nonmilk coffee lighteners be used?

These substances usually have considerably more calories than real milk. They are made from a variety of vegetable oil products, and in all of them various chemicals are used as stabilizers, preservatives, coloring agents, and so forth. Worst of all, many of these lighteners are made from vegetable oil products that are heavily hydrogenated and highly saturated and cause elevation of one's cholesterol. The fact that the label says that there is no milk in a lightener does not mean that it is safe for you from a cholesterol standpoint. Many people who are on cholesterol-controlled diets are very badly misled by these nonmilk creamery products. *If you have a cholesterol problem, do not use any of them without the specific approval of your physician.*

Is there any objection to sweeteners in coffee?

Sugar is never allowed. Artificial sweeteners without any calories are always allowed. Artificial sweeteners that come in powder form often contain lactose. This does contain calories. Do not use these sweeteners, therefore, except in cold beverages in which only the powder form will dissolve. Saccharin tablets usually do not dissolve in cold drinks.

Do not let yourself be trapped without saccharin. Your hostess or restaurant may not have any, so always bring your own.

How many calories are there in the artificial sweeteners?

There are no calories in pure saccharin or in cyclamates. As mentioned above, however, some artificial sweeteners are marketed, usually in powdered form, that contain lactose—a milk sugar. This has as many calories as any other sugar. Since most of these packets contain enough lactose to supply about 3 calories per serving, three to four packets of them a day adds about a pound of body weight per year. Check the labels and avoid this extra pound by not using these artificial sweeteners except for cold beverages or cold cereals that require sweetening, but in which saccharin tablets would not dissolve. There are some forms of saccharin, marketed in liquid form, which do not contain any calories. But read the labels carefully; if the brand contains sorbitol, it may have as many calories as the artificial sweeteners containing lactose.

How safe are the artificial sweeteners?

At this time, cyclamates are not considered safe and therefore the government has forbidden their use but their safety is being reconsidered. They have a great advantage over saccharin in that they are more stable to heat and dissolve somewhat more easily in cold beverages. Their heat stability is particularly advantageous when they are used in the manufacture and processing of canned or bottled foods and liquids. Cyclamates also have a less bitter aftertaste than does saccharin. I personally have not been convinced that cyclamates are dangerous, and do not object to their use in moderation, but I would not recommend them in the face of the government's edict. Incidentally, in some people (possibly one out of eight) cyclamates undergo a different form of chemical decomposition, which may be why some individuals object strongly to their taste and use.

Saccharin, too, at this time, is considered somewhat suspect by the U.S. Food and Drug Administration. In the more than 50 years that saccharin has been used, I am unaware of any harmful effects from it. I do not object to its use by my patients, but, at the same time, one must not be blind to any new discoveries about its safety, or rather lack of safety.

If these artificial sweeteners are not as safe as originally presumed, I am sure the danger would be related to the quantity used. Accordingly, the prudent individual will certainly avoid their excessive use. It is very difficult to define excessive use precisely. So far as the artificially sweetened dietetic beverages are concerned, I suggest restricting their consumption, as previously mentioned, to no more than two 16-ounce bottles daily.

As this is written, new artificial sweeteners are being planned which will probably appear on the market shortly.

How does one avoid the bitter aftertaste of saccharin?

Some persons are more sensitive to this than others. If you are particularly aware of this aftertaste, there are two things that you can do. First, avoid the cheaper forms of saccharin and ask your pharmacist for one of the better brands. Quality does show through in saccharin.

Second, the most bitter aftertaste develops from the decomposition that results from heat. Therefore, in hot beverages such as coffee or tea, do not add the saccharin until you feel the beverage is cool enough to drink.

Is there any problem in using sugar substitutes if you are gassy, or intolerant to milk?

Anyone who fits this description should avoid sugar substitutes containing lactose (milk sugar). Read your labels! If you are a sugar-substitute user, and are forever gassy, try going without them for a while.

What is sorbitol?

Sorbitol is technically an alcohol which is made commercially from glucose. It is the most common substance used to give a sweet taste in dietetic foods, and has been particularly advocated for diabetics who must avoid sugar. Its advantage to diabetics is that it is metabolized so slowly that it does not affect the level of glucose in the blood. But it *is* absorbed and metabolized and ultimately yields as many calories as does sugar. As a dieter, it is calories you are concerned about, so beware of sorbitol.

19

Wines and Liquors

If alcoholic beverages are part of your life style, there is no objection to including them with your diet, within appropriate limits. You should not give up food for alcohol, but rather always remember that the alcohol is an extra, over and above your diet. The more you drink, the slower your weight loss will be. The addition of one alcoholic drink per day to a normal diet will result in a weight gain of approximately 1 pound per month. Simple arithmetic will show that a nondrinker who does not change his eating habits but adds one alcoholic drink per day will have gained 12 pounds by the end of the year! The dieter who drinks alcoholic beverages should realize that he will lose weight more slowly.

Why isn't alcohol included in the Diet Plans?

Alcohol is not a food and therefore cannot be included in the Diet Plans. It is allowed in appropriate amounts, which will be defined later, because for many people it is an important part of their life style. I do not advocate the use of alcohol, nor do I object to it. Mostly, I permit it for the dieter.

What is the relationship of alcohol to appetite?

For centuries it has been known that a small amount of alcohol is an appetite stimulant. A large amount of alcohol will do two things: On the one hand, it can dull the appetite, but it may also make you not care whether you stick to your diet or not. Therefore, it is important to avoid excesses of alcohol while you are on a diet. This is in addition to the calories in the alcoholic beverage itself.

How much alcohol should the dieter allow?

Over the years, I have explored many different formulae, and have found the following system the most successful:

When possible do not drink.

Save your drinking for those social and business occasions where it is most important.

Anticipate your alcohol needs so that you do not use up your entire allowance early in the dieting week.

Men should restrict their drinks to seven a week.

Women should restrict their intake to a maximum of three drinks per week inasmuch as their caloric requirement is less than men's. Though this restriction may seem to be unfair, the formula has worked quite well.

May the drinks be taken together, or must I have them on separate days?

I do not think it matters if you space your drinks on different days, or find it more comfortable to drink a few at one sitting and then none for a while. How you space your drinks may depend on your particular social needs as well as on your own mood, but do not exceed the quantity allowed for the week.

What is the definition (portion size) of a "drink"?

Ale or beer—8-oz. glass (not a 12-oz. can)

Brandy—1½-oz. jigger

Champagne—3- to 4-oz. glass

Sherry—2-oz. glass

Whiskey (bourbon, gin, rum, rye, scotch, vodka)—1½-oz. jigger. Incidentally, if you have had whiskey on a plane, this is the size of the miniature bottles served.

Wine—3- to 4-oz. glass

Are there any alcoholic beverages that should be avoided?

Do not use sweetened wines, sweet vermouth, or sweet liqueurs or cordials.

May I have mixed drinks?

Mixed alcoholic beverages very often contain added sugar or sweetened wines (red vermouth) or liqueurs. A whiskey sour, even though called a sour, contains sugar. Some mixed beverages have no sugar, but by custom are served in quantities too large to be considered *one* drink. Martinis are typical of this group.

May mixers be used?

There is no objection to the use of water, unsweetened soda water (club soda), or the carbonated diet beverages. Avoid ginger ale (unless dietetic), tonic water (unless dietetic), sweet soda, or most fruit juices. Tomato juice may be used.

Which whiskies are lowest in calories?

The differences between different whiskies in respect to calories is so infinitesimal that unless an individual were measuring his portions with chemical pipettes, it would scarcely be perceptible.

Is beer more fattening than whiskey?

If taken in proper amounts, it does not matter whether you drink beer or whiskey. Remember, though, that the correct beer portion is an 8-ounce glass, not a 12-ounce can or bottle.

Doesn't wine have fewer calories than whiskey?

Ounce for ounce it does, but a wine glass holds 3 to 4 ounces as compared to a 1- to 1½-ounce whiskey serving. Therefore, glass for glass, the calories are the same.

What is the best alcoholic beverage if you want one low in alcohol content?

Try dry vermouth. Have it on the rocks with a lemon peel, or mix it with plain soda water.

What are the best wines for the dieter?

In general, only dry (table) wines should be used when on a diet program. The sweetened (dessert) wines have too many extra calories.

Is there any difference between white, red, or rosé table wines?

Not for the dieter.

May I use wine in cooking?

Yes, but if it is more than a 2-ounce portion per person, consider it as part of the alcohol allowance.

How do you handle an insistent host?

Let him pour and serve the drink. No one says you must drink it. In fact, at most parties the host is usually concerned whether his guests have drinks in their hands, not whether they are drinking them!

If you have had enough wine, the universal signal when your host is pouring more wine is simply to hold your finger on the top of the glass.

How do you make a drink last longer or "go farther"?

Mix it with a large quantity of club soda or water. An engineer I have treated told me that the way he stretches a drink is by ordering a type of whiskey he does not like and mixing it with club soda (which he says he hates): though he is acting sociably, he barely finishes his drink.

A very good trick is to say you are very thirsty and before you have your drink ask for an accompanying very tall glass of water. If you fill up on water first, you will be less likely to gulp down your drink. This was a trick taught to me by a professional tennis player, who always did this after a game of tennis to keep from overindulging in liquor merely because he was thirsty.

May I have sangria on a diet?

No. Sangria is a Spanish wine-fruit mixture with added sugar. It is really a high-calorie, sweetened, alcoholic fruit punch, and not appropriate for the dieter.

Is it permissible to have more than the allotted number of drinks under special circumstances?

Most persons can hold their drinks down to the Diet Plan allowances of three for women and seven for men. Under special circumstances, I allow women to increase their drinks to six or seven a week (vacation is a good example of a special circumstance). At the most, I would allow men one or two extra drinks during the week.

What can be done if my social schedule or business requirements make it impossible to keep my drinks down to the allotted amount?

If you feel the social pressures are so great that you are unable to restrict the alcoholic beverage intake to the allotted amounts previously stated, then I would strongly suspect that alcohol is truly a problem. I have often used the term *mini-alcoholic* or *junior alcoholic* to describe this type of person and feel that in many instances this reaction is symptomatic of the onset of true chronic alcoholism. Many social drinkers are unaware that they are in an early stage of alcoholism. I say this, not to offend, but rather to warn those individuals who constantly have excuses for why they exceed the weekly alcohol allowance. Going without alcohol one day does not insure that you are dealing adequately with alcohol. If you fall into this category, the very best thing that you can do for yourself is to stop drinking completely—NOW!

What may the dieter nibble on when drinking?

Only raw vegetables if available. Otherwise, nothing.

20

Food Preparation for Weight Control

The Diet Plans are all based on the rule that all cooking must be on a nonfat basis. Butter, margarine, lard, cooking oils, or shortening are never allowed, not even a dab. This does not mean that this will hold true after your correct weight is achieved, but it does hold true for the present!

The basic problem with cooking without fat is the tendency of meats (especially veal, chicken, and fish) to dry out. Beef and lamb will broil well with a high heat if cooked briefly, but veal, chicken and fish do best if cooked over low heat for longer periods of time. The difference in the cooking techniques that give best results arises from the fact that there is less fat in veal, chicken, and fish, and the protein fibers are of shorter length, whereas the reverse is true of beef and lamb. The use of aluminum foil, or of *covered* cooking utensils, will help tremendously to retain the moisture in these meats and avoid drying them out.

Cooking with wine is also a good method for diet cookery. This does not mean drenching the food with wine, but rather using it as a flavoring device.

Now let us consider the questions dieting patients most often raise about the cooking of their food, and explore this highly important aspect of any weight-control program in more detail.

DIET COOKING OF MEATS

What is "diet sautéing"?

This is the name I have given to the method of placing the food to be cooked over a bed of mushrooms and/or onions. Both these foods add flavor and since they have a very high water content, they will substitute for the usual fats used in sautéing. But do use a covered skillet!

What is the best method of basting in diet cookery?

This question always gives me a chance to pass on a valuable basting technique well known to French chefs: Never baste with cold liquids. Cold basting will bring the fluids of the poultry or meat to the surface (the same principle used in getting bloodstains out of cloth by the use of cold water), and may result in its drying out. Hot liquids help to congeal the protein and seal the liquids in (again, the same principle that explains why you never use hot water to remove a bloodstain).

What is the best way to prepare meats for the Diet Plan programs?

Meats may be broiled, boiled, steamed, baked, roasted, or stewed. The *best* way of all is to broil them over an open rack. The open rack may be of the type one uses on a charcoal grill, or an insert in a broiler pan that allows the fat to drip through. Some dieters purchase fluted, throw-away, aluminum foil pans which allow the meat to broil and the fat to collect in the channels. Pan-broiling, however, allows the food to fry in its own fat, and is therefore less desirable.

May breading be used if I do not eat the bread at lunch?

No. The Diet Plans are designed to create an eating pattern. Arithmetical calorie substitutions often inhibit the learning of proper eating habits, the development of which is usually best accomplished by repetitive techniques, with as little variation as possible. Incidentally, breading often requires some type of fat to hold it to the food.

What is the best way to prepare chicken?

The same rules hold true as for the cooking of meat. Frying or sautéing are never allowed. Use heated lemon juice, tomato juice, consommé, or clear soup stocks for basting. Remove the skin from chicken before cooking, as it contains much fat.

May one fry chicken if the skin is not eaten?

No, because the fat does seep through. Because of the fatty nature of skin, it should not be eaten, even if the chicken is broiled.

Is there any good diet stuffing for poultry?

I do not know of any that are not very high in calories. Avoid all stuffings.

DIET COOKING OF FISH AND SHELLFISH

What is the best way to prepare fish and shellfish on a diet program?

One starts with the premise that butter, margarine, and breadcrumbs are not allowed at all. Therefore, frying fish or shellfish is out of the question, unless it is done on a Teflon (or similar-type) pan, or with lecithin spray mixtures for frying, without added fats. Fish and shellfish (especially clams, oysters, etc.) can be eaten raw, steamed, poached, boiled, baked, or broiled. Obviously the form of cooking that is most desirable often depends upon the type of fish or shellfish being cooked. Marinate in milk, lemon juice, lime juice, or tomato juice. Consommé can be used for basting, but, as previously noted, never use it cold; heat all basting fluid *before* pouring on the fish. A small amount of wine yields a lot of flavor and the alcohol will evaporate in the cooking. Or try cooking fish or shellfish on a bed of onions and/or mushrooms as described above. Use covered pans and a low temperature. Be willing to experiment a little bit and if one recipe fails, keep on trying!

Boiled lobster really does not have to be dipped in melted butter, steamed clams can be dipped in clam broth, and oysters are tasty without breading. Soft-shell crabs can be broiled; they do not require sautéing.

May I use cooking aids of the "Shake and Bake" type?

No. They contain fat.

DIET COOKING OF VEGETABLES AND FRUITS

What are the best ways to prepare vegetables?

Vegetables should be cooked without any fat or oil. Flour or cream may not be added for thickening, nor may they be glazed with sugar or honey. Basically, all cooked vegetables are to be boiled, steamed, or baked. Avoid overcooking to save both flavor and vitamins.

Are cooked fruits allowed?

Yes, they are. The important consideration is that they be cooked without sweetening. If you wish to sweeten, use artificial sweeteners and add them after the cooking process is completed.

DIET COOKING OF EGGS

What is the best way to prepare eggs?

Eggs may be prepared by boiling or poaching. They may be soft- or hard-boiled according to taste. Some people are able to scramble eggs without fat by using extremely hot skillets, but I have never been successful at it. Eggs may be fried in a nonstick, coated pan or in a regular pan treated with lecithin spray.

May one fry eggs or other foods using lecithin spray mixtures?

There is no objection to using these substances for frying. They are available in spray cans and only minimal quantities are used.

What is diet French toast?

Diet French toast is simply a slice of bread soaked in a mixture of egg (the right number from your Diet Plan) and skimmed milk from your allowance and fried in a nonstick skillet. Add some artificial sweetener and cinnamon for taste.

OTHER DISHES

What are diet pizzas and diet Danish?

Diet pizza is simply a slice of bread, cheese, sliced tomato and spices, baked in the oven. A diet Danish is cottage cheese on a slice of bread, sprinkled with some cinnamon, and baked in the oven. There is no objection to either of these for breakfast or lunch so long as the quantities are in accordance with your Diet Plan.

What is the best way to make a grilled cheese sandwich?

Basically this is a melted-cheese sandwich. Using the amount of bread and cheese called for in your Diet Plan, it is simply a matter of melting the cheese on the bread in the oven, but without butter! If you order this in a restaurant, tell the waitress "No butter!"

In the final analysis, there are definitive limitations on cooking and food preparation. It may be difficult to be a gourmet on these Diet Plans, but there is no reason why you cannot fully use your ingenuity and imagination to create interesting, tasty, and imaginative meals without straying one bit from the Diet Plan.

Part Three

OBSTACLES AND INSIGHTS

21

The Stages of Weight Control

There are four basic stages in weight control: the initiation of the program, the "long-pull" stage, the drop-out stage, and the maintenance stage.

The initiation of the program. The ease or difficulty of this stage depends upon the strength of one's drive or motivation. The individual who is not fully motivated to lose weight tends to find the beginning of a diet difficult, but it gets easier as he gets used to the program and is rewarded by the early weight loss. Most individuals, however, usually start with a high degree of motivation and drive. They instantly develop the feeling that "nothing can stop me." They, too, are rewarded with high weight losses at the beginning. Gradually, the amount of weight lost each week lessens, often culminating in no weight loss around the third week, which I have named *quitter's week,* ushering in the second stage of weight control.

The long-pull stage. This is the period when the initial enthusiasm has worn off, when one encounters plateau weeks in spite of following the diet, when one begins to resent the self-denial being endured, when the goal still appears quite far off. This is a major period for drop-outs because of a basic lack of stick-to-itiveness. It may be a reflection of the type of diet the individual is on, particularly if it is a diet not very compatible with his style of living. It may be due to a lack of motivation, or to a return of some of the patient's psychological needs that made him fat to begin with. Or it may simply be boredom! Sticking it out is certainly a measure of your self-felt *need* to be thinner.

If you are having trouble at this stage, stand in front of a full-length mirror, as suggested previously, and stare at yourself, preferably without clothes, or possibly wearing an old dress or suit that you still can't wear with ease, and ask yourself if you are thin enough. Ask yourself whether being thinner still isn't worth the price of self-denial.

Few dieters can go through stage two without running into a few blocks: a social event that one simply cannot handle adequately, or a trip, or a holiday, or a personal annoyance that is dealt with by eating. *All is not lost.* Each of these events should simply be regarded as a confrontation. If you fail, simply restart from that moment on. Those individuals who hit a problem, handle it poorly, and then use it as an excuse to stop dieting, invariably regain all their weight so that someday in the future they must again begin the entire dieting process. For most people, dieting involves a series of confrontations.

I like to describe these confrontations as being similar to climbing over a high wall. If you fall down, the only sensible thing to do—assuming you *want* to get to the other side—is to pick yourself up and climb again. And if necessary, again and again. If you quit, you are saying in effect, "I do not want to be thin."

There are few dieters who do not have to overcome these confrontations. You can do it, that is, only if *you* choose to do so!

The drop-out stage. The third stage occurs just a little short of the goal, often when one is seemingly making no mistakes. This stage of dieting is often the most discouraging. Many years ago I ran a "failure section" in one of my Health Department clinics. By grouping the patients who had either failed to achieve a proper weight, or, more often, who had achieved it but could not keep it, I came to some very interesting conclusions after a long period of study. Most failures had two things in common: Either they did not have any supervision during maintenance, or, more often, they never completed a program to achieve their ideal weight but rather stopped before reaching their goal. *It is essential to proper maintenance that you go all the way to reach your correct goal, and not quit a few pounds too early.* It *is* worth the agony, if that is what it seems like to you. Because so many of the reasons for stopping short of your goal are psychological, it is especially important for a dieter in this stage to study the psychological questions discussed in Chapter 23.

The last stage, of course, is keeping to your new weight when you have reached it. The paradox of this is that though the vast majority of dieters have the most trouble with this stage of dieting, it is the one about which the least is known and the least is written. There has hardly been any research in this area. The large rate of failure in dieting is mostly a failure in maintenance.

One of the reasons why maintenance has been so difficult is that many people have dieted in such a manner that they never learned an eating pattern they could rely and build on to develop permanent, sound eating habits that were nutritionally and culturally correct for their life style. If you return to your old habits of eating after a diet, you will obviously return to your initial weight. Maintenance depends on the permanent learning of new eating habits. In addition to this, sooner or later most dieters must come face to face with the extent to which they use eating, overeating, and overweight as psychological tools. Lastly, you must accept the concept that though maintenance does not mean perpetual dieting, it does mean lifelong control.

The various questions that tend to arise in relation to the *stages of weight control* will be discussed on the following pages.

Why do people lose more weight at the beginning of a diet?

The first week of a diet (almost any diet) is usually characterized by a dramatic reduction in calories from previous levels as well as a reduction in salt. The naturally occurring salt in food is lessened inasmuch as the amount of food is lessened, and there is also less food to which you add table salt. The decrease in salt results in a large outpouring of fluid through the kidneys (medically this is known as diuresis), sometimes enough for you to awaken from sleep a few times each night. This large, early weight loss is therefore mostly water.

Is it necessary to take diuretics (pills to get rid of water) to get the diet started?

I strongly suggest that no diuretic be taken without a specific prescription from your physician. They are certainly not necessary to begin a diet. The use of diuretics should be restricted to specific medical conditions (hypertension, etc.) as diagnosed by your physician, or for the control of excessive premenstrual discomfort.

What is "quitter's week"? Why does it occur?

To me, quitter's week is a week in which people are either tired of dieting, or the scale does not show an adequate weight loss, so that they reason, "what is the point of dieting if I am not going to lose enough weight." This usually occurs around the third week of the diet. Most people, as noted above, though not all, lose most weight in the first week of a diet, somewhat less the second week, and often none the third. The extra weight loss in the first week has usually more than compensated for the lack of loss in the third week, but most dieters become rather emotional about this lack of loss, decide to stop dieting. If one merely persists in the diet, quitter's week is usually followed by a resumption of weight loss. A word to the wise dieter should be sufficient. There is no need to quit.

What are "plateaus"?

Plateaus are any length of time in which there is no measurable weight loss on the scale. They may last a few days, a week, or even a few weeks. The most common plateau is that occurring in the third or quitter's week.

Are there any other plateaus in dieting?

Yes, there are. Certainly most women will retain some fluid a week before their menstrual periods. Their weight may even go up. A small percentage of the women I have treated have a reversed pattern and retain water immediately after their periods rather than before. These are typical, recurring plateaus.

There are also plateaus that are caused by an increased salt intake. Some people who get bored with dieting will try to compensate for the lack of quantity by intensifying the taste of food. One of the most common methods of doing this is by using more salt. The increased salt will often cause some water retention, and an apparent weight plateau.

Every now and then dieters do reach plateaus for unknown reasons, but invariably the plateau period stops and people will go on to lose weight. Do not allow a plateau period to disturb you. It is extraordinarily rare for one not to break through a plateau if one is willing to stick it out. If you cannot break through, do not be alarmed, but see your physician. You may be obtaining calories or salt from some unrealized source, or possibly are taking a drug that may be resulting in water retention.

What is the best way to break through a plateau?

Ask yourself the following questions:

1. Are you nibbling without realizing it?
2. Are your foods being prepared differently (with added oil or by frying)?

3. Have you increased your salt intake?

4. Are you taking any new medication that may be causing salt retention?

5. Have you increased your alcohol intake?

6. Are you using marijuana and letting "the munchies" get the best of you? *If none of the above hold,* then

7. Are you as careful with your portions as you were at the beginning of the diet? *This is the most common cause of plateaus.*

If none of the above is the cause, keep a diet record for one week. Record your weight at the beginning and the end of this period and show it to your physician. (If there is a loss, it is not a plateau.)

If you are in a plateau period and then take an appetite-depressant pill, what should be expected?

Obviously, if you begin to lose weight after taking an appetite-depressant pill, it means you are eating less. This makes one's diet prior to the diet pills somewhat suspect. You must have been eating more than you realized.

What is the best way to weigh myself? Are some scales better than others?

Ideally, the best scales are those of the balance-beam type, but these are expensive, probably too expensive for home use. If you would like to buy one, it will certainly cost you over $50. Ordinarily the standard, spring-type bathroom scale is more than adequate for the dieter. These scales are subject to rust because most bathrooms are quite humid; also, the tension on the spring will change with the passage of time. But for most purposes, these scales are perfectly adequate to use to weigh yourself. Incidentally, very few scales work well on a rug, so keep your scale on a hard, level surface.

When is the best time to weigh?

Most people have found that the ideal time to weigh themselves is in the morning, on arising, after they have gone to the toilet, before breakfast, and before getting dressed. This is, of course, the most consistent way of weighing. Actually, it does not matter when you weigh yourself: before meals, after meals, morning, noon, or night. The important thing is to be consistent and to weigh yourself at the same time of the day each day, wearing approximately the same amount of clothing.

How often should I weigh myself?

Actually, if you are on a diet, I do not think that you should get weighed more than once a week. I think the tiny ups and downs are much too confusing, falsely encouraging or falsely discouraging. Simply weigh at the same time, once a week.

22

Occupational, Social, and Travel Problems

Early in any diet, you soon discover that certain events in your life style make dieting considerably more difficult. Just what do you do when you are invited to dinner for the first time by a new daughter-in-law? Or at a party where you are meeting the hostess for the first time? Or on a train, or a plane, or at a resort, or camping, or in a foreign restaurant? What do you eat when your friends suddenly surprise you with a party? This list, unfortunately, could go on and on, with each situation a difficult one for the dieter to deal with. For many of these dilemmas there simply are no rules to go by. You can only use your very best judgment.

When you are in a food trap, first ask yourself if it is still important for you to get thinner. If this is the case, you must then figure out how you can stay as closely as possible on the Diet Plan without insulting your hostess or those around you. Once in a while there is no choice but to go off the diet. If, however, you are constantly telling yourself that there is no choice, then you are psychologically choosing not to get thinner and are using these events as an excuse. Restaurants should rarely present a problem inasmuch as you have your choice from a menu. Do not be afraid to ask your waiter for assistance. The more you ask, the better service you will probably get anyway. Demanding people generally are taken care of the best.

Be a little sly. Don't be afraid to invent a few excuses, such as that you have an upset stomach and are being very careful, or that you have an allergy, or are seeing your doctor the next day "for tests."

Don't hurt your new daughter-in-law by not tasting the chocolate fondue—but a taste can be very small! If you have a difficult lunch situation at work, bring lunch with you. You are always sure of having a correct meal that way. If you are going on a long driving trip, stop for meals before you get overwhelmingly hungry.

In all circumstances, use your head.

How do you diet on trips, planes, tours, vacations, etc.?

Planes. Today, planes probably have the best portion control of any commercial food units I know. There is no such thing as a large portion on a plane. Therefore, you never need to worry about the size of their portions. Many of the foods served are high in calories, so you must pick and choose among what is on your tray. Invariably, the dessert is a high-calorie sweet. The airlines have learned that a sweet dessert is a psychological substitute for larger main-course portions. Eat your main course and avoid any high-calorie, sugar-sweetened fruits and cakes. Take the salad without the dressing. Scrape the sauces off the meat. If you are flying first class, you may feel that the only way you can get your money's worth is by eating everything offered to you. For this reason, you had better not travel first class if you are on a diet.

Many airlines provide special diet meals which may be ordered in advance.

Trains. There is less and less long-distance passenger travel on trains. Those trains that travel long distance routes, of course, have dining cars. Use your own judgment in dining cars: You have a menu so you have a choice. The choice you make will depend on how badly you want to become thinner.

If you are a commuter, stay away from the bar car.

Hotels. Hotels in general are of two kinds. Those with large à la carte menus should not be a problem to the dieter. Dieters who are at resort-type hotels whose rates include meals (American plan) do face a problem. If you believe that in order to get your money's worth at an American-plan hotel you must eat as much as possible, then I suggest that you do not go to this type of resort if you are truly interested in dieting. But if you use your good judgment, the hotels of this type very often have menus with a large selection. The larger the selection, the more likely you are to find something that contains the correct number of calories for your diet, and is good tasting.

Restaurant dining. In general, I like restaurants because they offer people a choice of foods. Do not be afraid to express your wish to your waiter. He is being tipped for his service so there is no reason why you cannot ask him for service that meets your needs. If you want something made in a special way, ask in advance. He will tell you if it can be done or not. It is not his fault if you do not ask beforehand and then after it is brought say that you really meant to order it without butter. You do the asking—first.

Foreign restaurants. There is no objection to a dieter eating in foreign restaurants. You can go to an Italian restaurant and not eat pasta or to a French restaurant and not eat thick, rich sauces. We could list restaurants of every type and description, but frankly the restaurants that cause the largest problem are the ones which serve Chinese food.

The problem that dieters have with Chinese food is that most Chinese restaurants use a large amount of oil in the cooking. Though prepared in a wok (the traditional Chinese cooking utensil), in a sense most of their food is fried. Many of their foods are thickened with cornstarch and sweetened with molasses. Most Chinese foods are also accompanied by rice (occasionally fried) and noodles (almost always fried). Chinese food is basically too high in calories and is often thirst-provoking because of the large amounts of salt or monosodium glutamate used in the cooking. Although it is filling at the time of eating (because of the large vegetable bulk) one is hungry again soon afterward because of the often meager protein content!

I strongly advise that you stay away from Chinese restaurants in the early stages of a diet. If you must go, order only steamed items such as steamed vegetables, steamed shrimp, chicken, lobster, fish, and so forth, and specifically state that you want the oil and the cornstarch left out. Certainly eat no rice or noodles.

Vacations. Many people on a vacation often feel a kind of release from responsibility. However, you must approach your diet in the same manner in which you approach your other health needs: If you go on a vacation, you do not run away from good health practices. You do not forget to take a toothbrush just because you are going on a holiday. If it is important to you to lose weight, *bring* your diet with you. There is no reason why you cannot have a happy vacation and be thinner too.

Official banquets and wedding dinners at restaurants. The problem with these affairs is of course that there are no choices. These are fixed meals. You must decide whether to eat each item that comes to you. If it is extraneous, if it is unnecessary, if it is the wrong food, avoid it unless it is a main course. If it is a main course take a half portion, and scrape the gravy or other sauce away. In the final analysis, your desire to be thinner will establish how much you will eat at these events. As previously suggested, at those official parties where many appetizers are served, the large trays of hors d'oeuvres are often well decorated with raw vegetables, and you can eat these garnishes. They are food, and very low in calories.

Coping with Thanksgiving, Christmas, Passover, Easter Sunday, and other holidays. The important concept here is not to make them eating orgies. The idea is not to see how much food you can stuff down and still survive. There is no reason why one cannot have festive foods and enjoyable holidays within the framework of a diet. To walk away from a table saying, "If I had another bite, I would burst," is an insult to one's health.

What can be done about being extremely hungry when going to a very late party?

Parties that are very late, so that there is a long stretch between your afternoon snack and dinnertime, may present a hunger problem. Handle it by eating your evening snack just before you go to the party. Add a salad and a glass of milk to that and you have what I call a small meal. Two hours later, when it is time to eat at the party, you are not ravenous and do not feel as if you could devour everything in sight including the tablecloth. Of course, you will not have a late night snack since you will have eaten that before you went to the party.

How do you cope with aggressive hostesses who say, "You must try this. I made it especially for you," or "You can start your diet tomorrow. Don't diet when you're here"?

The answer to this starts with knowing your hostess—and how well you can resist her pressures. Then just invent an excuse. In most instances, the easiest way to deal with the situation is to take the food that is offered, but leave it on the plate, without eating it! Play with it; move it around the plate. In my experience, the aggressive hostess is much more interested in what you put on your plate than what you eat. So take the food and let it remain there if it is the wrong food. She will not be insulted by this, and probably will not even be aware of it; she is mostly concerned that you take some of it. Just give the appropriate thanks and say how good it tastes. If that is not enough, tell her you are allergic, or have a digestive problem.

What is a food trap?

A food trap is a situation where only the wrong food is served or is otherwise available. I divide food traps into two kinds: primary and secondary. A primary trap is one in which you are served a main course that is totally wrong and for which there is no substitution. This is handled simply by taking a half-portion. Usually, that is enough to make it relatively harmless from the calorie standpoint. The secondary food trap occurs when a food not on your Diet Plan is served to you as a nonessential part of the meal: For example, if potatoes are served, simply do not eat them.

How do you control binges?

By never letting them happen! If you don't cheat the first time it is impossible to cheat the second time. If you feel an uncontrollable urge to devour all sorts of food, do not think you can handle it by a taste. This simply opens the door to an orgy. Instead, change what you are doing. Go for a walk. Go into a clothing store where there is no food. Go to the barber's. Get a shoe shine. Take a hot bath (a great way to stop the desire to break the diet). Basically, do something physical and something different. And do ask yourself how much you want to be thinner.

How do you handle "cravings"?

I do not think there is anything physiological about cravings. I believe cravings are a matter of wanting something that you are not allowed to have, simply because it is forbidden. Craving is really just saying, "I am not allowed to have this; therefore I want it and I'd like to blame it on some biological reason." People find it ridiculous to think they would ever crave raw vegetables, yet most travelers who go to Mexico and are afraid to eat raw vegetables usually begin craving salads. They may not even like salads usually, yet now they crave them. Upon returning home where raw vegetables are available, they no longer crave them. I know one person who rarely ate bacon. On going to a hotel that did not serve it, this individual, not liking the hotel, immediately began fussing because he could not have bacon. The answer to craving is really to ask yourself how important it is to get thin, how badly you really want to reduce. If you truly want to be thinner, you'll realize there is no such thing as an irresistible craving. Do not magnify the term *desire*.

If you really want to eat more, what should be done?

I guess the most important thing here is to ask yourself whether you want to be thinner or fuller. If you want to be fuller, the answer is to go ahead and eat; if you want to be thinner then the answer is not to eat, unless it is the correct eating called for in your Diet Plan.

How do you make up for errors on a diet?

There is no such thing as making them up. This is where many people get into trouble. If you make an error on a diet, ignore it and simply take your next meal in the normal way called for by your diet. Do not eat less because you ate more the meal before. This simply starts a round-robin series of events of eating less, eating more, eating less, eating more, etc. Break this pattern by eating the correct amounts, even though you feel that you can eat less and so make up for your previous lapse.

What is "the rubber band theory"?

This is the name I have given to the method of coping with mistakes on the diet. Regard your diet as a rubber band. No matter how distorted a rubber band becomes, when the tension is released it will revert to its natural shape. Consider your diet in the same manner. No matter what errors are made, let the next meal be an exact diet meal. Do not try to compensate by eating less or differently. Do *not* try to make up for mistakes!

What is the best way to deal with guilt feelings after making a mistake in dieting?

The best way and the only way, as just suggested, is to ignore them and restart the diet with the very next meal. What is done is done. The important part of dieting is dieting, so get back to it immediately.

How do you avoid wasting food on a diet?

Start out by never preparing more food than you are entitled to eat. There is no need to cook a whole package of frozen food if your Diet Plan calls for only a part of it. Why can't you cut the frozen package in half, continue to freeze half, and prepare the other half?

The one thing worse than economic waste must surely be the biologic waste—the net medical result of what happens to you when you weigh too much.

Do circus fat ladies have glandular problems?

Believe it or not, extremely obese people are usually simply big eaters. Many years ago when I was serving my internship at Bellevue Hospital in New York City, we had a patient who was a professional circus fat lady. Unfortunately she had severe high blood pressure and was told that unless she lost weight she would probably die. She was put on a hospital weight-reduction diet and did lose a little over 100 pounds. But she faced a tragic dilemma. During her hospital stay she became more and more concerned with the fact that if she lost much weight she would lose her job and her ability to support herself. One night she developed a bronchial asthma that was extremely unresponsive to treatment. After many difficult days with her asthma, she was told that she had lost enough weight. Miraculously, her asthma stopped. She began to eat more and she retained her job in the circus world, but soon died as we had feared she would.

23

Psychological Problems of Dieting

As anyone who has dieted knows, the course of dieting is never smooth. It is beset by traps inadvertently set by hostesses, and traps set by being at the wrong place at the wrong time. But most of all, one sets his own traps, and these all too often turn out to be self-made psychological traps. As much as people blame restaurants and parties for their fatness, most fatness develops in your very own home. The list of these self-made psychological traps goes on and on, and the questions which follow are those asked most frequently about them.

What is the significance of dreaming about food or dieting?

This probably means that you are more concerned about your need to diet than you realized when awake. It does not mean that you will be a better or poorer dieter.

I have heard some funny dreams about dieting. One patient told me of a dream in which she imagined she was taking a shower, but when she turned on the shower all that came out was cottage cheese!

What do you say to people who say you have lost too much weight?

This is a matter of knowing people. You can discuss it with some people, but with others you cannot. If they are the latter sort, agree with them, and then when they ask why you are still dieting tell them you are not dieting, but simply learning maintenance. It is pretty tough for anybody to come up with an answer to that one.

It is interesting to notice just which persons tell you you have lost too much. Occasionally they are relatives who are concerned that perhaps your weight loss is from illness, and not from voluntary weight reduction. They require reassurance, often quite frequently.

Friends, co-workers, schoolmates, and distant relatives often tell you that you have lost enough weight. More often than not, these are people who are overweight themselves. One of the most annoying things to many people is to watch someone successfully achieve a self-disciplinary effort. They are often really jealous or envious.

What is a verbal cop-out in dieting?

By "a verbal cop-out" I have in mind one of those words that lets you get away with something that you know is incorrect. For example, a "sliver" of cake. All dieters eat only a sliver of cake. As a matter of fact, I think the word "sliver" is used more with cake than it is with anything else. This is a verbal cop-out. It is as if you got away with eating the portion of cake by calling it by a diminutive name. There is *no* cake on a diet. You should not eat it on a diet.

Other verbal cop-outs are, of course, such expressions as "just a taste." Remember, it is still just a taste too much. If the item does not belong on a diet, it should not be tasted.

If your spouse suggests, in a restaurant, that you try a bit of the particularly choice entree he has ordered, the odds are that you already know how it will taste, and you should take his word for it that it is good. The excuse that one must taste when one is cooking is often another of these verbal cop-outs. But the biggest one of all in dieting is the phrase, "But *I* don't eat that much!" The point is that if you are not losing weight, or staying within your correct weight, you are eating too much *for you*.

Is there such a thing as unconscious eating?

There certainly is. I once had as a patient, a middle-aged schoolteacher who was going through a period of much anxiety because of problems related to her children. One day, at a point where her anxiety was at a particularly high level, she was preparing a sandwich to take with her for lunch. After making it, she stopped to do something else, and then when she was ready to leave and take the sandwich with her, looked around for the sandwich and could not find it.

She knew she had just made it but simply could not find it. Finally she went into the bathroom to brush her teeth and there was a piece of lettuce between her teeth! She realized then, that without being consciously aware of it, she had eaten the sandwich. This is what I mean by unconscious eating. It can readily be controlled by forcing oneself to be aware. Similarly, unconscious eating sometimes occurs during sleep-walking. I have had a patient tell me that she knew when she went to sleep at night, there was a full container of ice cream in the freezer. When she woke up in the morning, she discovered that the container was partially empty and since she lived alone, she had to be the one who had eaten it during the night without realizing it. She said that she would have blamed her cat but unfortunately, her cat did not know how to open the freezer door.

If one wants to lose weight, isn't he motivated?

I think there is a huge difference between desire and motivation. Desire, in this case, is wanting to be thinner, but this may simply be a fantasy wish, like that of the teen-ager who wants to be a movie star and daydreams that when she goes to bed at night she will wake up in the morning and find herself in Hollywood. This, of course, is a classic adolescent fantasy. But compare this to a girl of the same age who also wants to be a star, but takes acting lessons, goes to the auditions, attends all theater that she can. She is more than desirous; she is motivated. In other words, she is willing to do do whatever is necessary to accomplish her goal. This is motivation. There is a vast difference between the dieter who merely wants to be thinner, and the one who will do everything necessary, no matter how severe the self-denial, to accomplish the goal of thinness. I ask all my patients who are having difficulty losing weight to evaluate their true motivation, not simply their desire.

Do some people stay fat to avoid sex?

Absolutely. As suggested earlier, many persons who deep down are afraid that they cannot cope with the sexual demands of the people they go out with, or even of their spouses, keep themselves fat in order to avoid appearing desirable to the other sex. This is usually on an unconscious level, and the patient often vigorously denies it at first. Sometimes thinking carefully about the unconscious tendency will enable people to realize that this may be the reason why they are fat. If this is your problem, you may need some professional help. If you discover, after losing weight successfully, that you are not handling this problem adequately, and if under the stress of increased sexual demands you are beginning to regain weight, do consult your physician.

What are the chief psychological reasons for going off a diet?

In my experience the chief reason for going off a diet is eating in response to anxiety or tension. Sometimes the anxiety may appear to accompany a depressed state, but true depression, as in the grief after loss of an immediate member of the family, is more often associated with loss of appetite. The cause of anxiety may be serious worry, as in problems with the health of a child or parent, or fear of loss of a job, or other financial crises. The anxiety may be associated with school work or problems with a boy friend or girl friend. Regardless of the cause, *most overweight people deal with their tensions by overeating.* You can deal with this in two ways. You must first confront the cause of the tension directly and try to resolve it. Second, you must ask yourself whether the eating will actually help the tension. Of course it will not. To say that you do not care about losing weight is certainly untrue, for though you may not care at the moment, you will surely care the next day. But if you upset your diet now, it will be too late tomorrow to correct the damage. Care in time. Think out your problems and tensions carefully. The more you can deal with them on an intellectual level, the better off you are.

If the tensions are overwhelming and unresolvable, then you must teach yourself to keep your eating divorced from your emotions. Remember, no matter how upset you are, care is still taken in watching out for traffic as you cross a street. Ask yourself, when you are eating today, if you will be happy about it tomorrow.

How do you keep from eating because of boredom?

If boredom is truly causing excessive eating, then the most obvious thing is to try to fill your time more productively. *Force yourself* to do something more interesting. Instead of feeling sorry for yourself, do something. Find a hobby for yourself. Paint, do sculpture, sew, knit, or play a musical instrument. Do something, especially with your hands. Most people with boring lives create this boredom for themselves.

Do people stop losing weight because they are afraid of being successful in life?

Believe it or not, this often happens, as in the case of an actress patient who kept saying that when she lost weight she would certainly land good roles. By never getting thinner, she avoided the confrontation. If you begin to slip in your dieting, or find yourself making more and more mistakes, ask yourself whether possibly you are afraid of giving up your favorite excuse and no longer being able to avoid meeting a final challenge.

In many ways people may be truly afraid of coping with life with slim figures. My advice is to try coping. Most likely, you will be successful and will be much happier. After all, you can always get fat again if you so desire!

Some people say that they do not want to lose weight because they probably will regain it. Is this true?

If you expect to regain weight, you probably will. But this is a copout. You do not have to regain it if you do not wish to. Yes, I said wish to! Sooner or later almost every one of my patients has heard me say: *"Every time you put the wrong food in your mouth, you are choosing to be fatter, while every time you put the correct food in your mouth, you are choosing to be thinner. Being thinner is entirely a matter of your choice."*

What does morality have to do with dieting?

I have always wondered why so many dieters go around calling themselves "good" or calling themselves "bad." It is almost as if they are looking for a tremendous amount of approval and backslapping because they have dieted correctly, or, on the other hand, are looking for some type of punishment because the diet was not followed correctly. Rather than looking for punishment, a little bit like George Washington when he cut down the cherry tree, if you confess you assume absolution follows. I do not consider gaining weight, or losing weight, as an issue in morality. I would much prefer, and I have always suggested to my patients, that they should see themselves as dieting correctly or incorrectly, and wipe out the concept or morality in dieting. Adherence or nonadherence to a diet, though it is a measure of one's self-discipline, does not really make a good person or a bad person.

I have many middle-aged or older patients who are highly respected leaders of their communities, often with very large financial or governmental responsibilities. It certainly sounds silly to hear an ambassador come into my office and announce, "I've been a bad boy," referring to his failure to adhere to his diet. When people make an error in their dieting, I try to persuade them to say they were incorrect, not bad. The significance of this is simply that to get thin and stay thin one must have a fully mature approach to the problem. This is one of the reasons why it is so difficult for youngsters to reduce. They often simply have not achieved the maturity necessary for success. Adults require this maturity also.

Should you tell your spouse or parent what you weigh and how much you lose each week?

I do not think so. On the other hand, I do not think that you should lie either. Sooner or later the change in clothing size becomes obvious, and when one is losing weight successfully, it is hard to exclaim at each weighing how much you have lost. Do not pressure a child to tell you his weight. It just adds more tension. As I said earlier, sooner or later the changes in your appearance and in the fit of your clothes will speak for themselves.

Does food ever serve as a substitute for sex?

Very often. Sexually frustrated people often head directly for the refrigerator for a different kind of fulfillment.

Does dieting increase libido (sexual desire)?

Many patients, both men and women, have told me that as they got thinner they had a greater sexual drive and interest. This is probably due in part to better health, but is mostly the result of feeling better about themselves—what the psychiatrists call "increased ego." People do respond to their own attractiveness and, of course, their mates almost always do. Positive responses from your mate in turn reinforce your own responsiveness.

What can be done about loss of libido on a diet?

This is an unusual event. It is rarely the result of the diet, but usually the result of some other psychological factors operating at the same time. In some cases the same lack of libido was present when the individual was fat, but was hidden by the thought, "Things would be different if I were thinner." Many people feel that dieting and getting thinner is the answer to all their problems, only to find after successful dieting that many of their problems are still with them. Being thin is not the answer for all ills. *In fact, getting thinner sometimes uncovers problems rather than being a panacea for them.*

Do fat people have difficulty having sexual relations?

There are very few problems that are insurmountable when it comes to sex, and fat is not one of them. Very few overweight people complain that this is a problem, even though the fatter two people are, the more contortions are sometimes necessary. Many people wonder when they see a couple in which the man is excessively overweight, and the woman quite tiny, how she is not injured when they have intercourse. In these situations, the women usually assume a superior position, or they use a lateral (side) position.

Are fatter men more virile?

Men of larger size are no more virile than lean, scrawny men. Sexual abilities are unrelated to body size.

Do fat men have large penises?

No, they do not. In fact, in men who are enormously overweight, the genitals are often partly hidden by abdominal and suprapubic fat, making them appear smaller rather than larger.

How many calories will sexual intercourse use up?

Statements by other authors notwithstanding, probably very little. In spite of the fantasies of many people, the actual sex act is usually quite brief. In general, women exert less physical activity in the sex act than do men and therefore expend fewer calories. Excessive sex may be fun, but it is hardly a substitute for dieting.

Are homosexuals ever overweight?

Male homosexuals are usually very aware of their bodies and very sensitive to unattractive features. In general they are quite careful about their weight control, but obesity is sometimes seen in homosexuals, though not commonly.

Obesity occurs in about the same percentage of female homosexuals as among other women, but the former tend to seek help for it less often.

What is behavioral therapy and what is its relation to external and internal cues?

All humans respond to certain physiological events, such as an empty stomach or lowering of the blood sugar, by a desire to eat. These events have been called *internal cues*. We all also respond to *external cues*—the appearance of food, the time on the clock, a type of social event, and so on—which also promote a desire to eat. Many psychologists believe that overweight individuals have an increased responsiveness to the external cues. Perhaps this is why some overweight people say they are never hungry but can eat all day long. Yet people can control these desires, as is evidenced by the large number of overweight individuals who will not eat in front of others.

Some psychologists feel that if an individual were taught to associate certain types of eating with unpleasant things or events, it could act as a negative control. Ultimately, however, all changes in eating style are in a sense behavioral changes. As I have said earlier, the only way one will learn to be thinner is by teaching oneself a new style of eating, developing a new conditioned reflex pertaining to appetite and its control. But unlike some of the modern behaviorists, one must recognize that human beings have a lot of thinking power (the psychologists call this *cognition*). I believe behavioral patterns can be changed best on a rational, thinking basis—a basis of insight and understanding—and not on an artificial association of overeating with unpleasant things. The basic association must be, simply, that overeating makes fat.

Why do diets fail?

Usually it is dieters, rather than diets, that fail. In fact, some 80 to 90 percent of dieters fail either to achieve a correct weight or to maintain that weight. If we except children, there are indeed few first dieters. We can classify almost all dieters who have failed in one or more of five categories; only one of these groups fail because of the actual diet they chose to lose weight by. The five chief causes of failure are as follows:

Lack of desire. These are the many people who start diets but are not really desirous of being thinner. You see this particularly in children, unimpressed with the need to lose weight, and in many older person who decide that there are enough things in this world that they can no longer enjoy, so why should they also give up the pleasure of food.

Diet education reasons. Many individuals are not successful basically because they have never learned the rights and wrongs of eating. Failure for this reason is becoming less common with the advent of the large number of diet clubs throughout the country. The most significant contribution of these clubs is in the education of the public in valid concepts of how to eat correctly to lose weight.

Cultural reasons. Some people change their minds about losing weight for cultural or social reasons, which are often actually insufficient to justify abandoning one's diet. Thus, for example, a man may wrongly feel that if he loses any more weight he will no longer seem virile, or a woman may begin to fear that she will lose all her curves and no longer look feminine.

Metabolic problems. I believe this to be the least frequent reason for failure. In my own experience of over 20 years in this field, I have found that less than .01 percent of failures were for metabolic reasons, and even those cases were difficult to prove. Although there have been many articles in the medical literature as to why diets fail for metabolic reasons, I am personally unconvinced that this occurs.

Psychological reasons. This is the most important reason why dieters fail. The psychological reasons that make people overeat in the first place are the same reasons that come back into force during the diet to make them go off it. These people tend to overeat under tension, under anxiety, out of boredom, as a weapon against parents or spouses, and so on. When the psychological reasons for the overeating recur, they may take precedence over the desire to be thinner.

24

Medical Complications While Dieting

Dieting is essentially a medical experience. It results in physiological changes in the body. These changes have been the subject of many questions asked by my patients, which I shall answer in this chapter.

Is it safe to leave fats out of a diet?

First, let me answer this by saying that it is almost impossible to leave all fats out of a diet. Fat is present in so many foods that it is extremely difficult to bring down our caloric intake from fat to less than 20 percent. It would also make our diets highly unpalatable. It almost requires formula diets to achieve the extremely low fat intakes.

There is enough fat in the most restricted diets to supply the essential fatty acids required by the body. In the even more modern diet planning of today, we are concerned also with the type of fats; saturated or polyunsaturated. *Saturated fats* have been implicated as a cause of increased atherosclerosis (hardening of the arteries) through the elevation of cholesterol levels in the blood. The opposite is true with *polyunsaturated fats,* which appear to be able to lower cholesterol levels in many persons. Today, the vast majority of physicians advocate the use of low-fat diets, with as much fat as possible being polyunsaturated rather than saturated, as a safe method of weight reduction. Only in infants (children under 2 years of age) is there some question about fat restriction and the need for essential fatty acids.

Will a low-fat diet cause dryness of the skin?

Not in my experience.

Do fat people have worse skin than others?

Not necessarily, but I have made one special observation. Many overweight people have very thick, dry skin over their elbows that begins to clear as they lose weight. I do not have an explanation for this but believe it is related to a condition called pseudo acanthosis nigricans. The condition is not considered common, but in my practice, it is not unusual.

Does dieting cause skin changes?

Mostly, the changes are favorable. Many dieters note that their skin appears clearer on a good diet. Occasionally, one develops a rash, which is usually the result of an allergy to a food being more frequently eaten on the diet than prior to it. If this is the case, begin a series of food eliminations. Start with fish, the shellfish, then citrus fruits, tomatoes, and then the other foods until you establish which item is the offender. Eliminate each item for a full week before going on to the next item.

How can I prevent my skin from getting "crepey" as I lose weight?

The degree or the amount of wrinkles and the degree of crepiness will depend on a few things. It will depend to a large extent on your age. Obviously, children do not have wrinkled faces while older individuals do. I have always felt that people who have had excessive amounts of sunlight tend to have an increased amount of skin wrinkling. There has been a recent report that smokers get more facial wrinkles than do nonsmokers. But the most important thing is probably how stretched with fat the skin has been over a long period of time. The longer the skin has been stretched, and the greater the degree of stretching, the less likely it is that the skin will bounce back. After a while, one has to truly raise the question whether it is worth losing more weight if the wrinkles continue to be more evident. I think this is a decision that only the individual concerned can make. In some situations plastic surgery can be done with remarkable results. Massage and exercise will not tighten stretched skin.

Will I lose my stretch marks after I lose weight?

No, not really, unfortunately. But what happens to stretch marks is that with the passage of time they get fainter and fainter. Stretch marks are probably due to a breaking of the elastic fibers in the skin. Once these fibers are broken there is no way to put them together again. These torn fibers show as stretch marks. Stretch marks are rather common; women who have had children almost always develop them on their abdomen. With the passage of time, however, there is a gradual fading of the stretch marks, and though in general they do not disappear, they will usually become hardly noticeable, even though they are very noticeable when they are new, having a purplish look. An unusual amount of stretch marks, or stretch marks with very minimal weight gain, warrants an investigation to check on the possibility of endocrine disease.

Does milk keep one's face from getting wrinkled?

This is an unfounded rumor. Skimmed milk is a good food, an important food for the dieter, but it does not have any magic properties to protect the face. A well-rounded, nutritious diet is what gives the skin a good texture.

Since I started my diet, I have noted my skin getting yellow. What does it mean?

If the whites of your eyes are yellow also, it has nothing to do with the diet, and probably means you are jaundiced. See your doctor immediately.

If the whites of your eyes are still clear white, but the remainder of your skin is yellow (best seen in the palms), you probably have the condition known as carotenemia. This results, as previously mentioned, from the excessive ingestion of carrots, pumpkin, and other orange-colored fruits and vegetables. The condition is usually harmless and simply requires elimination of the orange-colored produce. Some people are more prone to this condition than others. The reason for this is unknown.

Can dieting cause any change in the fingernails?

The diets outlined in this book will not cause any harmful effects to the fingernails. If you have soft and splitting fingernails it is probably not diet related. Detergents used for dishwashing are more often the cause. I would suggest that, rather than change the food in your diet, you use the brush-on nail hardeners that are found in cosmetic departments in many stores.

Can gelatin be used to stop splitting of fingernails?

I do not believe that gelatin helps prevent splitting nails. If you insist on eating gelatin, use the unsweetened types of plain gelatin. If sweetened, it must be the diet type that is artificially sweetened.

What can be done for excessive amounts of falling hair?

Though occasionally blamed on dieting, a well-balanced diet high in protein (as are the Diet Plans) will *not* cause hair to fall out. The reason for excessively falling hair is unknown. Occasionally it is attributed to hormonal changes, and occasionally it is benefited by the use of thyroid hormone. Consult your physician about this. He, in turn, may refer you to the hairdresser, but it is nice to know you do not have a serious medical condition causing hair loss.

Can dieting make you shorter?

This sounds like a silly question but it is based on a very interesting patient of mine. I had treated an 18-year-old boy who came to me weighing 469 pounds. Over a 2-year period, he lost 284 pounds, coming down to a weight of 185 pounds. Out of curiosity, he asked me to recheck his height at the end of the program, and to my amazement, he lost a half inch! I had seen older persons who became somewhat shorter as the years went by, but I never saw anyone get shorter at his age! Of course I rechecked his height. I decided that he had simply lost fat from his scalp and from the soles of his feet. Thus I came to the conclusion that one can get shorter on a diet, but one would probably have to lose over 200 pounds!

Why do I look tired on a diet?

Probably because you are not getting enough sleep. I did not say that in jest. The major blame for fatigue on a diet may be placed on the diet, but this blame would be misplaced unless the diet was deficient in carbohydrate. Those diets that are very low in carbohydrate (the *energy* nutrient) often do cause fatigue, but this is not true of the Diet Plans in this book. The Diet Plans will not cause fatigue. Lack of sleep will. Incidentally, when one has an insufficient amount of sleep, one often gets irritable, and there is a tendency to break the diet. Protect yourself! Get enough sleep!

How can I avoid getting a very thin face during weight reduction?

One of the first complaints that dieters have is that people are telling them that their face is getting too thin. The answer to this is that they are probably not getting too thin, but getting thinner. After all, all of us are accustomed to recognizing people by their facial appearance, and it is rather easy to notice if someone has lost the merest millimeter in his face. At the same time, we might not notice if someone had lost an inch or two around the waist. We are accustomed to looking at people's faces and not at the circumference of their waists. Consequently, people are quick to notice facial changes. In my experience, faces do not become as thin as people think they do. And if they did, there would be no reason why one could not get accustomed to having a thinner face. Lastly, it is my experience that after maintenance there seems to be an adjustment of some of the fat back to the face, and the thinness of the face is less noticeable. I do not know why this is true, nor can I explain it, but it is an observation repeated many times. I do not think that a thinner face should be an excuse to stop dieting.

As an afterthought, some of the people who say your face is too thin may just be a little envious!

How can I lose weight in my hips, in my thighs and in my rear, but not anywhere else?

Frankly, you cannot. There is really no way known to modern medical science on how to spot reduce. *Spot reducing* is the term that we use for losing weight on one part of the body and not any other. The body has no capacity to take weight off in one area and not in another. A crude example possibly would be to try to visualize a method whereby the body could take weight off the left buttock and not off the right. There is no special food, there is no injection, there is no medication that I know of, or that any established medical scientist really knows of, that will allow you to take fat off one part of the body and not the other.

Fat can, however, be hidden, and the trick to spot reducing is the trick of hiding fat. There are three ways to do it. The first is through *exercise,* which tightens muscles. By tightening muscles, or by adding tone, as we say medically, we become firmer. This pulls in the fat to make it appear that there is less there. There is no actual loss of fat inasmuch as the fat is above the muscle layer, nearer to the skin. Another way of hiding fat is by *posture.* After all, if we spread the amount of body weight over a few more inches, one must look thinner. Whether you are sitting or standing you will look thinner by having good erect posture. Stand taller, sit taller, and look taller and thinner! Do not underestimate the importance of this. Still another way of hiding fat is by the *use of proper clothes.* Women discovered a long time ago that girdles helped to control a bulging abdomen. The style of your clothes can also make a significant difference. It is obvious that some clothes will make one look thinner, and other clothes make one look fatter. The broad big plaids will make one look fatter, whereas thin vertical stripes often make people look thinner. But do not spend your life trying to camouflage fat. Instead, lose weight.

How do you avoid "losing" your bosom on a weight-reduction diet?

Obviously, if a woman is going to lose weight she is going to lose some of it in her bust. Very often women would rather lose it all from the hips and not from the bust, but this is impossible. *There is no way to lose fat selectively.* If one wants to lose more weight below the waist, one must put up with losing some weight from the bust and possibly other areas of the body.

Are there any special diets that will allow you to lose weight where you want it?

Believe it or not, all, *yes, I said all,* diets do this. Think of the psychology of the statement. Overweight people usually want to lose weight where they have most weight, and most weight is always lost where one has the largest amount of extra fat tissue. Therefore, one loses most weight where one most needs reducing. Do not misinterpret this statement as a pitch for fad diets. You always lose weight where you want to, but you cannot stop losing weight where you do not want to—no matter what diet you are following.

What is lipodystrophy?

Lipodystrophy is simply the medical term for uneven fat distribution. There is no known cause or cure for this. An extreme of this is a condition called *steatopygia* in which there is enormous fat accumulation in the buttocks of women of some African tribes.

Why is it so difficult for many women to lose weight below the waist?

It is really unknown why those women with excessive amounts of weight below the waist appear to lose weight more slowly than those with fat accumulation in other areas. Weight *can* be lost from heavy thighs if one is persistent enough and willing to put up with "getting there on a local train instead of an express"! The need is for persistence.

What do you do if you notice that your legs get swollen while on a diet?

The first thing you should do is see a physician. Until your appointment with him, eliminate all table salt and any naturally salty foods.

Occasionally, I get a swollen joint, particularly in my large toe when I go on a diet. What should be done?

This sounds like a typical case of gout. Persons with gout may have a tendency to have an attack under stress of dieting. See your physician about this.

Does dieting affect one's menstruation?

Occasionally, dieting may change one's menstrual cycle, with the development of some irregularity. Adolescents and young women who have lost a significant amount of weight will often have their menstruation stop altogether. Medically this condition is known as *amennorrhea*. It is not serious, and apparently as the body adjusts to the new weight and a new style of eating, menstruation will return.

Do fat people have trouble conceiving?

All fertility specialists advise their overweight patients to lose weight. Of course, they advise other things also, and what gets the credit for causing eventual conception is not always clear. People who lose weight become more attractive and usually think better of themselves. People who think better of themselves tend to function better and this is probably equally true in the sexual areas.

If I have an upset stomach, must I eat everything on the diet?

When your digestive system is not up to par, and you therefore have a much smaller appetite it is ridiculous to force yourself to eat more. I would simply suggest that you eat less, but stay within the form of the diet. The Diet Plans outlined are rather bland, and are more likely to help a digestive problem than aggravate one. If there is a period of indigestion, eliminate roughage: raw vegetables and raw fruit. Avoid these for a day or two. There is no objection to eating cooked vegetables and fruits, but do not exceed the allowed limit. If the indigestion continues or gets worse, by all means see your physician.

How does one control constipation?

Constipation is the most common complaint in dieting. It is primarily the result of the lack of fat in the diet. Inasmuch as fat acts as a natural lubricant, the less fat the less lubrication, and the more likelihood of developing constipation. Fat also serves as a stimulant to bile flow, and less bile promotes constipation. If you have constipation, deal with it by an increase in raw vegetables and make sure that you are taking a full quota of raw fruit. However, if you become gassy from this increase in raw fruits and vegetables, cut down your intake of these foods, increase your noncaloric fluid intake, and, if necessary, use a mild laxative. Incidentally, if you eat less there will naturally be less fecal bulk and obviously you will have to move the bowels much less. Do not be alarmed about constipation, no matter how regular your habits were before the diet. Constipation should be treated only if you are uncomfortable.

Prune juice and fig juice should be avoided because of their high-calorie content. Sauerkraut juice helps some people, but its salt content is high.

Should my diet change if I develop diarrhea?

If you develop diarrhea, do the following. Stop all roughage. Eliminate all raw vegetables and raw fruits, and use only cooked foods. Stop drinking milk, but maintain a high fluid intake. Use one of the simple medications from your pharmacy. If your diarrhea persists, or if you develop fever, see your physician.

What do I eat when I have a cold?

First of all, do *not* load yourself up with fruit juices. There is nothing curative about fruit juices. Fruit juices do supply additional vitamin C and are a source of fluids to counteract the dehydration that often accompanies fevers. If you have a cold and have a rather listless appetite, stay with the Diet Plan but eat smaller quantities. Maintain a high fluid intake, but use the low-calorie fluids such as iced or hot tea, iced or hot coffee, or skimmed milk (from your daily allowance). You may use the low-calorie diet sodas, but do not drink *extra* fruit juices.

If you wish, each fruit on your diet may be replaced by 4 ounces of unsweetened fruit juices, but watch the limit! As I said earlier, there is nothing curative about fruit juices. If you prefer, or your physician suggests that you have an extra amount of vitamin C, take it by tablet. Vitamin C tablets (also called ascorbic acid) are over-the-counter preparations and relatively inexpensive.

What may be taken for a cough?

If you have a cough, avoid syrupy cough medicines. Most of them have a very high sugar content and, despite the smooth feeling they give when swallowed, they have a minimal therapeutic value, not significant enough to make up for the extra calories in the syrup. The same is true of lozenges. If your cough persists, or you develop a fever, by all means see your physician. Let him prescribe for you but ask him if he can give you a cough medication that is in tablet form and therefore noncaloric. There are very effective prescription items available for cough control in tablet form.

I have been using honey for a cough. Will that ruin my diet?

Of course it is wrong for your diet. It is just an extra, unnecessary source of sugar. There is absolutely no curative effect to honey. It is not soothing to the throat. In fact, if it did cling to the back of the throat it would simply be additional food for bacteria to grow on!

Is it safe to have a surgical operation when one is overweight?

The answer to this really depends on how important the surgical operation is, in proportion to the extent of the overweight. Obviously, if one has an acute emergency (such as an appendectomy) that requires immediate surgery, there would seem to be no question as to the course of action, regardless of other conditions such as overweight. On the other hand, if one requires an operation that is not of immediate urgency (e.g., the repair of a hernia), most surgeons and anesthesiologists believe the less overweight one is, the safer are both the surgery and the anesthesia. Therefore, many surgeons will suggest to their patients that they lose a certain amount of weight before they go for the elective operation.

Why do I eat when I am tired?

I call this the "feed-fatigue-and-get-fat" problem. It is not clear whether this is a physiological or psychological reaction. But certainly many many people eat more when they are tired. There are three ways to prevent this. Awareness is most important. Be aware of the tendency to eat more when you are tired. Try to avoid eating anything that you are not entitled to on your diet. If you *must* eat, stay with the free foods such as coffee, tea, or raw vegetables. Most of all, use prevention. Avoid fatigue. Get enough rest and sleep on your diet. This is most important while dieting. It is false calorie economy to think you can burn up a significant number of extra calories by staying up later because this is usually overcompensated by eating too much. Instead, get enough rest. This prevents the extra calories resulting from feeding your fatigue.

Can you lose more weight by staying up later, that is, by sleeping less?

Theoretically, you should obviously use up more calories when awake as compared to when asleep. Therefore, the more hours awake the more weight lost. However, the compensation for this is that when you get tired there is a tendency to feed fatigue with food. And when you do this you get fatter, not thinner. Thus, you are much better off getting a sufficient amount of rest and sleep. When you do not have enough sleep you are irritable, less determined, and more likely to change your mind about continuing on your diet. Avoid fatigue and get enough sleep. It does help a diet.

How do you keep up with the clothing size changes as you are losing weight?

This is difficult. If one makes a big investment in new clothes too soon, it may act as a deterrent to further weight loss. I recommend to all my patients that as they lose weight they do not invest in new clothes, but have alterations instead. It is ultimately cheaper to throw out an altered garment than a new one. Some people have so much weight to lose that they must purchase new clothes as they progress. If this is the case, buy clothes as inexpensively as possible, as they may not fit you for long.

The longer you wait to purchase new clothes the better off you are. Even during the early parts of weight maintenance there is very often a further shift in body measurements that do change your clothing size. When you have lost a large amount of weight, you discover that almost every clothes item requires changing. This includes underwear, and even men's hats. I had one patient who lost 260 pounds, and at the end of the diet was able to fit the fingers of both his hands between his head and the band of his original hat! Even rings become too large, as do bracelets and wristwatches. When women lose weight in their hips they will notice that their skirts are getting longer, as men will notice their trousers look longer. In the same way, when one loses weight from the shoulders, blouse and shirt sleeves seem longer. The one item men should be most careful of is shirts. Neck sizes are quick to change, and a large shirt will provoke the comment, "You are getting too thin"—a nice comment but not necessarily a correct one.

In summary, I have never seen anyone who objected to buying new clothes because the old clothes were now too big for him!

Part Four

NONDIETARY APPROACHES TO WEIGHT CONTROL

25

Exercise, Massage, and Special Aids

Being *for* exercise in weight control is somewhat like being against sin—it is expected of you. I personally feel that the role of exercise is not particularly important in the treatment of overweight. In theory, the addition of any amount of caloric expenditure is certainly beneficial. In practice, I have found it almost impossible to get most of my patients to sustain an exercise program of sufficient magnitude to make a difference in their weight control program. The advantages and disadvantages will be discussed in the following questions. We shall also discuss in this chapter other nondietary approaches to reducing, such as appetite depressant pills, massage, reducing machines, steam baths, and others.

Should appetite depressant pills be used in dieting? Are they dangerous and if so why do doctors prescribe them?

The so-called appetite pills, which are really pills to take away one's appetite, are more precisely called anorexiants or anorectic agents. Most of them are fairly effective in reducing one's appetite. In some people they cause unpleasant side effects such as irritability, nervousness, palpitations; at times, fainting, and frequently insomnia. To avoid some of these side effects, some brands of pills also contain sedatives. Their most serious drawback is the danger of their being abused. The longer one uses these drugs, the more their therapeutic effect wears away, requiring higher and higher doses, which may not only increase the side effects but often lead to addiction or habituation. People who are depressed get a particularly good lift from these drugs, which adds to the abuse potential.

If taken for short periods of time, under proper medical supervision, anorexants do aid some people in dieting, and I daresay that many responsible physicians find them helpful in the treatment of overweight. *I do not. I personally do not feel that appetite-depressants are necessary or desirable, and, in fact, I believe they are a detriment in the long-term control of obesity.*

They often do take one's appetite away, but what happens when one stops these pills? Without appetite, how does one train appetite? It is like teaching a child to write without giving him a pencil. It cannot be done. One must learn to control one's appetite *during* the weight-control program. This is why the majority of people on pills regain their weight after they stop using the pills.

Some physicians say pills make it easier to get the patient started on a diet. Yet in my experience the most weight is lost, the most motivation is present, in the first weeks of dieting. I feel that at this time it is unnecessary to take pills.

A young, but very wise, patient of mine who said he "tried everything" to lose weight was discussing the use of these pills and made a very sagacious comment. He said, "You know, when I feel like dieting, the pills are great, but when I do not feel like dieting, they don't seem to work at all!"

What is the major purpose of exercise in weight control?

The major purpose of exercise in weight control is to contribute to calorie expenditure. The more activity, the more calories are expended, and the more weight one should lose. This, of course, is on the assumption that there will not be an increase in the intake of calories to compensate or even overcompensate for those calories lost through exercise.

Exercise has some distinct assets that are not related to weight loss. Most people get a feeling of well-being from it, and there is an accumulating body of scientific evidence that shows exercise to be highly beneficial to the cardiovascular system. Exercise also increases muscle tone, which, in turn, helps in figure control.

How effective is exercise in weight control?

Though most physicians take an opposite point of view, I do not think that *in practical terms* exercise is effective in losing weight. Exercise does burn up calories, which it does in direct relationship to how strenuous the activity is. You would use a large number of calories in chopping wood, much less in walking, and much less still in sewing. Obviously, for any given period of time, you use the most calories running, less in walking, less in sitting, and even less in lying still. When you consider that you would have to climb twenty flights of stairs to use up 80 calories (5 to 10 more calories than are found in a slice of bread), it is easy to recognize the very large amount of exercise necessary to lose a pound of body weight, which requires, as we have seen, an expenditure of about 3500 calories.

Thus, to expend a sufficient amount of calories to achieve measurable weight loss, a definite physical activity program would have to be embarked upon. I would have no objection to your developing and starting such a program, but just how practical is it? Describing an experiment in which a large number of calories are burned by a man chopping wood for an hour has little relevance to our culture. For effectiveness, any exercise program must be carried out on a regular basis. Often this is impossible under the pressures of our so-called civilized, rushing society. Walking is often cited as good exercise, but in our culture time is apt to be scarce. Unless we change our mores drastically, there is no possible way for most people to add sufficient exercise to their life pattern to make any appreciable caloric impact on their weight.

Are sports a good way to get exercise?

If you can add exercise to your daily schedule, it is beneficial. Sports are a nondrudgery method of doing so. But do get the full advantage, and do the job wholeheartedly. If you use caddies or golf carts, obviously you will use fewer calories than if you did not. Swimming is good, but you do not lose any calories while you lie on the beach. Obviously, every sport has limitations. And, of course, you must control your consumption of high-calorie snacks or beverages in response to the appetite and thirst consequences of strenuous activity.

What are the most effective exercises?

The most effective are those that can be done the most consistently. Some people are really quite physically oriented and never feel well unless they participate in some type of daily exercise. These are the individuals who, rain or shine, always find or make time for some regular physical activity. Most overweight (and many nonoverweight) individuals never seem to have the time for an exercise program. The best program for these people is an obligatory, enforced sports program. These may be enforced psychologically by paying money in advance to a gym and therefore feeling obligated to participate; or by enforced programs of physical exercise in colleges or in basic training in the armed forces. Few people can plan and carry out an effective program for themselves.

A convenient way of getting extra exercise is to add an *extra* mile of walking (as on the way to or from work or school) to your daily program. This is not enough to increase one's thirst or appetite and each mile will result in the utilization of 50 calories. Though there is not a *daily measurable* weight loss, such walks will result in the loss of a pound of body weight after every 70 walks.

Incidentally, the better the sportsman, the fewer calories are burned. For example, the better golfer walks less, swings fewer times, and spends less time looking for lost balls. The average golfer will burn about 400 calories after an 18-hole game of golf. The tennis player expends more calories per hour, but plays fewer hours.

What are the best kinds of exercise for persons who are not sports-minded?

Any type of walking is good, as is swimming. Supervised calisthenics or bicycle riding are also helpful. A fine exercise for women is dancing. Most Y's have classes.

Are increased appetite and thirst a significant problem after exercise?

The problem with increased hunger and thirst is not that they cannot be resisted, or be handled by eating and drinking correctly, but there is a tendency for the overweight individual to handle them poorly. A 12-ounce bottle of beer will add 170 calories, and twenty peanuts another 114 calories. That is almost 300 calories in a very short time. If you are thirsty, drink iced water, or the other noncaloric beverages.

Is exercise safe for everyone?

If you are excessively overweight, do not start any program without the permission of your physician. The older you are, the more important it is that you have professional supervision. Some people are better off waiting to begin an exercise program until they have begun to lose weight.

If exercise is so important to prevent overweight, why is it not important in treating it?

Lack of physical activity is not the only cause of overweight in our culture. Equally important is the fact that food is very abundant; convenience foods that are higher in calories surround us, and as we become more affluent we have more money to pay for this abundance. Also, we live in a culture in which all events are celebrated with food: holidays, weddings, parties, testimonials, and so on. Just meeting somebody in the street whom you have not seen in a long time often ends up by both sitting down with a cup of coffee and a piece of cake. The effect of exercise is not sufficient to counter that of affluence, food abundance, and fatty foods.

How often should I exercise?

As often as possible, but the regularity and consistency are more important than the frequency.

What is the role of massage in weight reduction?

Only recently, a young girl patient of mine explained to me that her mother had told her that as a young woman she had spent years getting her fat pounded away by a masseuse, and did not want her daughter to have to lose weight in such a difficult way. Well, in all honesty, one cannot lose weight from massage, not an ounce. There is no way to push weight off or on. Fat is in cells, cells with walls and nuclei, living structures in which the fat is chemically stored, and there is no way to push it out of the body physically. Passive exercise, which is the medical name for massage, may have some therapeutic values in people with muscular disease problems. Certainly many orthopedists advise the use of massage for particular muscle and joint diseases. Massage may make you feel better, but it will not help you lose weight.

What about massage for spot reducing?

No! As I said above, there is no way to push fat out through its cell walls. There is equally no way to push fat from the left side of the body to the right, or from the right to the left, or from top to bottom. There is no way to spot reduce by massage, no matter how much one gets pounded, squeezed, pushed, or rolled.

How good are various machines for weight reducing?

Machines fall into a few categories:

Vibrators. I call them the "fat jigglers" because all they do is jiggle fat. They jiggle it up and down, and in and out, forward, backward, and diagonally, but the fat is still there. There is no way to jiggle fat away. Vibrators have no medical value for weight reduction whatsoever. Nor do they have any advantage for spot reducing.

Rollers. These are in the same category as vibrators. Fat cannot be rolled or smoothed away. It is another exercise in futility.

Electric current machines. These supply small electric currents to various muscles and make the muscles move. In a sense this becomes an involuntary exercise, but the movement is really so small and so limited that there is no proved, significant, scientific, or long-lasting value to this type of machine for purposes of weight reduction.

The only exercise you are going to get from other electric-powered machines that do the work for you is that of bending over to put the plug into the socket.

The stationary bicycles. The bicycles are really a form of active exercise. It is a form of bike riding; you just do it in one place. I think what I said about exercise in general holds true here. The one advantage of these is that it allows one to use a bike in inclement weather and because of its ready availability it allows one to set up a daily schedule. This would enable one to do his exercise on a regular basis. Perhaps the only disadvantage to it is that on a nice day it is a shame that you cannot do this exercise outdoors and take advantage of the weather.

Gyms and weight-reducing salons. From the point of view of weight reduction all the gym can offer you is a place to do the exercise I have discussed previously. The reducing salons, of course, get involved with the machines and a lot of the beauty factors. I am not qualified to judge the beauty factors in the reducing salons, but I still do not know of any physical methods that can help you lose weight.

What is the value of the inflatable belts or wrappings in losing weight?

As I said earlier, fat is in cells with cell walls, and no matter how much compression you get from a belt there is no way to eliminate the fat from the cells. We do know that body tissue is compressible. Everyone knows the effect of a girdle, or the effect of wrapping a rubber band around a finger and watching the skin get compressed. Upon the release of the constrictor, however, the compression, of course, stops and the tissue returns to normal size. There is no scientific evidence whatsoever that any of these belts or wrappings, whether heated or unheated, cause any weight loss at all.

Are there any ointments or fluids that when applied to the body will take off weight?

There are none known to medical science. Absolutely none.

What about steam baths and saunas?

Steam baths and saunas will allow one to perspire and consequently lose water. If you lose water the scale will of course go down, and you will have lost weight. But the minute you get out of the sauna and have a glass of water, you will have regained the amount of weight you just drank. All steam baths and saunas can do is take off water weight. And water weight is immediately put on as soon as you drink the same amount of water, or other fluids. Inasmuch as there is a feeling of dehydration after a steam bath, you will drink back the lost fluid very quickly, so there is no effective weight loss. Remember, one must have constant equilibrium, constant balance between the faucet and the lavatory. One cannot lose fat tissue in any sauna or steam bath.

Part Five

BEING THIN ONCE AND FOR ALL

26

Maintaining Your New Weight

The goal in weight control is, not only to get to the correct weight, but also *to stay at this weight.* I have already suggested in the earlier section on the stages of dieting (page 175) that if, after concluding a diet, one returns to one's old style of eating, one will surely return to his former weight and the entire dieting procedure will have been useless. One purpose of the dieting technique is to get one down to the correct weight, but if the dieting technique does not also create a set of good eating patterns that become a habit, maintenance will last but a fleeting moment in time.

One of the paradoxes of weight control is that the majority of people who start diets do not maintain their weight, yet the majority of medical research is on how to lose weight, not how to keep it off! The experience with these Diet Plans has been that the majority of people can keep their weight off successfully and permanently. I carefully used the word *can,* because in the final analysis it is not the Diet Plan that is either a success or a failure. If you choose to be thinner, to accept the self-denial that goes with good dieting; if you are willing to change your eating habits permanently and to acknowledge that some of your eating may be in response to psychological needs and that you may have to adopt a different approach to these needs, then you, too, as so many others have been, will be successful. In the last analysis, you yourself must accept the sole responsibility for your performance.

I shall answer many of the questions that arise during maintenance, including those relative to the psychology of being thin, in the following pages.

Must one diet for the rest of one's life to be thin?

No, one need not. But one can and must expect to follow lifelong eating controls in order to remain thinner. Control does not mean dieting. We control how we dress, how often we shave or brush our teeth, or how we cross the street. In the same manner, one need not feel oppressively restricted if care and good judgment are used in food selection. Being careful does not imply the same limitations as does a diet.

Is it not safer simply to stay on the diet during maintenance?

If you did, you would continue to lose weight. There is truly no need to follow the diet during maintenance, but rather the need is to learn how to eat in moderation. It is something of a trial and error method, but the control is not difficult. There are bound to be some swings in your weight, but the method of having some leeway by keeping your weight a few pounds under the ideal is a most successful one. Do not be afraid to explore, but this never means giving yourself license to return to bad eating habits.

When should I stop dieting?

Not until you have gone two to three pounds below your correct weight. It is important that you have some leeway. It is extremely difficult to keep precisely at one weight. It is much more practical to hold your weight within a few pounds below your desirable weight. It will prevent the panic that otherwise accompanies a pound weight gain.

How restrictive must one be in maintenance?

After dieting properly and achieving a correct weight one can eat anything desired, but obviously not everything. There is a true difference between anything and everything. Most people can look in their closet and choose *any* garment to wear, but none can choose every outfit. In a like manner, with maintenance one should be able to choose any food, but never every food you might like at any one time.

Are there any other controls on maintenance?

Your clothing's looseness or tightness is always a quick indication of how you are doing, but during maintenance, it is not a substitute for daily weighing. Weigh at the same time daily, and remember, scales do not lie, only the people who read them! To avoid inaccuracy, do not place the scale on a rug, and above all, *do believe your eyes!*

What is the technique of number control?
My weight always varies from day to day.

The very best method of weight control is what I call the *traffic light system.* It is as near to foolproof as any I know. Establish your ideal weight and as I said earlier, get 2 or 3 pounds below it. Weigh yourself daily; if you stay below the ideal weight, I call this the *green light.* When the light is green you may go in any manner, or, in our terms, you may eat freely. Eat anything, but not everything. Use moderation at all times. So long as you are in the green light zone, continue to eat freely but carefully.

If you are at the actual weight you consider ideal, consider this the *yellow light zone.* Yellow means proceed with caution (not to stop, or in our terms, not to diet), but to be careful. If you go even 1 pound over the ideal, this is the *red light.* Danger! Stop! Go back! Go back on your diet and stay on it *until* you achieve the green light again. Do not wait until after the weekend! Do it now! *Dieting is not fun, but its results make life more fun!* And stay on the diet until you are back in the green light zone—2 or 3 pounds below the ideal weight.

What Diet Plan should I choose if I find myself in the red traffic zone?

Go back, very strictly, to the Diet Plan that you were following just prior to your achieving your ideal weight.

Are there any rules that should be followed in maintenance?

There are suggestions rather than rules. Most people have ended the diet enjoying the Diet Plan breakfasts and lunches. Many of my patients have suggested that they continue these Diet Plan breakfasts and lunches while on maintenance. The biggest need for more food, both socially and psychologically, is at dinner. That is the time to add some of the extra items you would like to eat. This does not mean going whole hog. Discretion is still the better part of valor. Have a starch or an extra portion, regular salad dressing, or a rich dessert—but not all of them at once. Make your food additions slowly and gradually.

If I eat more at dinner, what will keep me from gaining weight?

If you do not eat a little more during maintenance, as we have seen, you will continue to lose weight, so you should eat more. There is a major trick to avoiding gaining weight as a result. *For the rest of your life use fish, poultry, and veal for the main course in the majority of your meals. Continue to avoid—not totally but as much as possible—beef, lamb, pork, and pork products.* If you are willing to restrict these items, you will be amazed at how much spaghetti, potatoes, rich desserts, regular salad dressing, and so forth you can eat without exceeding your ideal weight. Of course, you must eat such foods in moderation. If you go back fully to the old, prediet style of eating, you will go back to your old, prediet weight.

The avoidance of beef, lamb, and pork is the single most important technique of permanent weight control. The more you rely on fish, poultry, and veal as main courses, the easier it will be to control your weight.

Which is the first food forbidden on the Diet Plans that most people choose to eat on maintenance?

Regular salad dressing is probably the first restricted food item to be reinstituted on the diet. There is no objection to this during maintenance, but the less fat and oil you use, the better off you will be.

Is there any objection if, in maintenance, I have milk shakes and cream in my coffee, and may I even eat French fries?

Yes, you may have any of these, but I think you will find most of these items rather rich for you. One really learns to enjoy a low-fat style of eating, after dieting according to the Diet Plans.

What is meant by "testing to failure"?

Some people eat a little more than they should, and note no weight gain. The next day they eat a little more again. This goes on and on until they eat enough to gain weight. If you have a successful way of eating, stay with it. Do not prove that with a little trying you can be a failure. The goal of maintenance is to eat more liberally, not to prove that if you ate enough, you would gain weight!

Is it true that no matter how thin fat people get, they always see themselves as fat?

This is often true, especially for people who were fat during adolescence. I have the impression that most individuals develop an image of what they look like during their adolescent years and maintain this image of themselves forever, no matter how they change in subsequent years. Psychologists have demonstrated this body-image concept in a variety of ways in people who have lost weight.

I have seen this so much that I call these individuals the "skinny fat person." They see themselves simply as fat persons "who happen to be skinny." This can be overcome. One can get a healthier and truer image of oneself, but it will take constant reminding. This body-image attitude need not be an excuse to get fat again.

Why does one gain so quickly when going off a diet?

Most people who go off a diet, do so excessively. After one mistake, the dieter often throws all caution to the wind, eats hundreds and hundreds (even thousands) of extra calories on a binge. Even when being extra careful on a diet, about all one can save is from 100 to 200 calories; thus, losing extra weight is a very slow process, whereas gaining weight tends to be very fast. Such is the unhappy consequence of human nature combined with caloric arithmetic!

How does one restart a diet?

I would simply start the Diet Plan today—not tomorrow. It is important that one should forget yesterdays in dieting. For some persons, a more restrictive program acts as a psychological boost in the beginning. If one desires this extra restriction, I would suggest the following, but limit it to one week only:

Eliminate all beef, lamb, and pork.
Avoid eating any ice cream.
Do not drink any alcoholic beverages.

Keep a careful, written record of what you eat. It is a reminder and does help. If necessary, get supervision from your doctor or from a diet club. And most of all, start *now*. It is *your choice* whether you wish to be thinner, and *your choice* how soon you wish to achieve the goal!

Index

ABOUT THE AUTHOR

Dr. Morton B. Glenn was graduated from the New York University College of Medicine and served his internship and residency at Bellevue Hospital. While working at Dr. Norman Jolliffe's Washington Heights Nutrition Clinic, he became especially interested in treating obesity. He succeeded Dr. Jolliffe as physician-in-charge of the clinic, then became head of the Morrisania Nutrition Clinic and Kips Bay Obesity Clinic of the New York Department of Health. A past President of the American College of Nutrition, Dr. Glenn has also served as President of the Food and Nutrition Council of Greater New York. Besides conducting a private practice in New York, Dr. Glenn is a Consultant in Medicine (Nutrition) at Knickerbocker Hospital and Assistant Professor of Clinical Medicine at New York University College of Medicine. Author of a previous book, *How To Get Thinner Once and For All,* he has contributed many articles to national magazines and professional journals.